Imbalance

The Perception of Unfulfillment in the
Modern Day Woman

DR. KATHERINE Y. BROWN

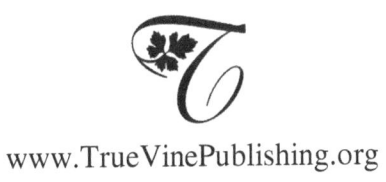

www.TrueVinePublishing.org

Imbalance
Dr. Katherine Y. Brown

Published by True Vine Publishing Co.
810 Dominican Dr.
Nashville, TN 37228
www.TrueVinePublishing.org

ISBN: 978-1-962783-10-1 Paperback
ISBN 978-1-962783-25-5 eBook

Printed in the United States of America—First printing

DEDICATION

To my mother, Roberta Baines-Wheeler. Thank you for always being the wind beneath my wings and for reminding me that my wings were meant to fly.

IN MEMORY OF

Little did I know when writing the dedication to this book that my mother would pass away just 24 hours later, on November 5, 2016. It serves as a reminder of life and the enduring love we carry for those who shape our journey.

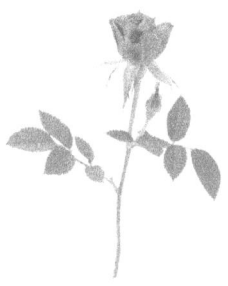

November 5, 2016

TABLE OF CONTENTS

PREFACE

In today's society, success is often identified by a well-defined completed checklist. Checklists include college degrees, affiliations with organizations, financial earnings, and more. But do these external markers truly signify success? Does it guarantee contentment and fulfillment from within?

Despite accumulating an extensive 30-page curriculum vitae, holding presidencies and leadership in top-tier organizations, and making appearances in newspapers and magazines, I felt a void, much like what you may be feeling or might have felt at some point in life. Contrary to what many expected, I stepped back from these roles, taking a pause to introspect. This personal journey led to a realization. As I spoke with thousands of women across different regions and backgrounds and the following recurring questions and themes surfaced.

- *Why did so many women claiming their family as a top priority fail to reflect this sentiment in the time actually spent with their loved ones?*
- *Why did some of the busiest, most outwardly successful women confide in me about their deep-seated unhappiness?*
- *Why did so many women, regardless of where they were from, express regret about repeating the same mistakes?*
- *What does it say about our definition of success when women, though celebrated professionally, struggle with self-worth internally?*

The common thread was imbalance. There was a common reported perception that despite having everything desired professionally, reports of being unfulfilled remained present. With these themes in mind, it must be clarified that the intent of this book is not to dictate the path women should take in order to achieve both personal and professional success. The purpose of this book therefore is to help the reader by encouraging self reflection and to provide a reminder that with every day there is the option to choose balance or imbalance. Select options that serve your desired outcome. There are no right or wrong choices because you are always in control to change your decision at any point. When we become aware of the power in having a choice, clarity happens.

I am committed to encouraging people to become the best version of themselves. My vision is to foster a space of healing, love, and respect for one another in our surroundings. The cornerstone of such a community is balance.

INTRODUCTION

Thank you for taking the time to open these pages. This book is for everyone, but especially those who are looking to make thoughtful and lasting changes in their lives. Although intentionally short and abstract in design, this is not a book that you should flip through rapidly. It is written to allow time for self-reflection and thought.

I want you to slow down and focus.

Ask yourself the questions provided as you read and honor where you are today in your life's journey. When you come upon a question, take a day to meditate on it and reflect upon your answers. Throughout reading this book remember to be kind to the person you were then, encouraging of who you are now, and optimistic about the version of "you" that you're creating. This was written with intent and the vision of helping you live a life of purpose.

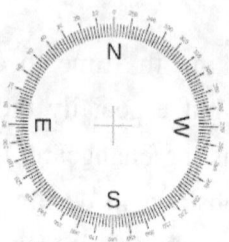

Life is about 360 degree turns and you are in control of pointing your needle in the direction that you desire to go.
Don't rush the process.
Be encouraged and empowered to slow down.....

To achieve balance there are times when you must slow down. Why is slowing down so important, you may ask? When you neglect your responsibilities or are scattered in thought, it impacts children, spouses, families, partners, the community, and you.

Most importantly, motherhood and nurturing are maternal instincts that shape the world. Women are encouragers and cheerleaders, but are often left in positions where their cheerleader pom-poms need to be shaken to encourage themselves. Asking for help is often viewed as a sign of weakness so many press on, pretending that all is well when in reality something is missing or they are struggling internally. Sometimes we know what is missing and sometimes we simply sense an empty void in our lives. When trying to slow down, some women perceive it as a lack of effort or an overwhelming feeling of not being enough. In efforts to uphold an image of strength, many respond by piling more tasks onto already full agendas. So I ask that you reflect upon the following questions.

What suffers when you don't slow down?

_____

_____

_____

_____

_____

_____

Who suffers when you don't slow down and take time for self care?

_____

_____

_____

_____

_____

_____

If you notice in the answers you put above there is always a sacrifice, the choice is yours. Regardless of your answers to the above questions, often those who love us most are the ones who suffer when we sacrifice ourselves. Sometimes we know the vicious cycle when it is occurring, yet we feel compelled to give in to the expectation that we must comply. To rationalize it, we tell ourselves, "Everyone does it" or "If I don't do it, who will do it" in an attempt to bring a sense of normalcy to our abnormal behaviors.

All too often, we live behind veils and facades and never let people know the obstacles we've encountered on the road we've traveled. When we do this, and others who observe us encounter obstacles, they feel as if they are alone.

They are not alone, and you are not alone. Life repeats itself in some way and sharing one's story can help empower another person to live the best life that they can possibly live. Your story matters. Your experiences are important and valuable. Always own and embrace your story, it is your truth. In doing so, this not only empowers ourselves but also inspires others. Sometimes, sharing experiences can help steer people away from duplicating the mistakes we made. At other times, it can reassure people of their positive path, encouraging persistence even when success seems distant.

Another part of your story may come from involvement in civic, social, faith based, and community organizations. As you participate in these organizations, it becomes equally important to remember that your worth comes from within. You are not validated by an organization! You are validated by you and not what you do.

Without this understanding you risk becoming imbalanced. When you are balanced, you avoid being in places and with people you are not aligned with. Be strategic, nothing happens by chance. If you are strategic in your business, you must be strategic with your life. And so this story begins...

Disclaimer: Nothing in this book should be misconstrued as medical advice. For any health-related concerns, always consult with a qualified healthcare professional.

CHAPTER 1:
SEEKING BALANCE

What exactly is balance? Sometimes the world seems to spin so fast at a dizzying pace that we feel a loss of control and powerlessness. We read self-help books and find few solutions with long-term, lasting effects in our lives. We want to be everything to everyone, yet this task can be draining.

With this context, it is important to define the discussion and focus of our conversation in this book. I am dedicated to a very specific kind of woman: a woman who is in a delicate place, at a crossroads, eager for transformation in thought, action, being and searching for a new way of thinking, doing, and becoming. This is for women who desire change but are uncertain of the steps to take or how to achieve change. It's for women with receptive hearts who may be fearful of breaking away from imbalanced societal norms that challenge their existence and purpose, yet have the desire to do so.

The solution you seek is already inside of you.

The quest for balance is a continuous journey, where the true essence lies in understanding oneself and navigating through life's complexities with grace and resilience.

At the end of this book, you will not look at any business meeting or endeavor the same. It is time for you to get tired of running around, symbolically beating your head against the wall in frustration, trying to be that which you are not, and winding

15

up either not recognizing the person you've become or not liking the person looking back at you in the mirror. This journey is a place for healing that encapsulates honesty, growth, and self-discovery.

IT IS TIME TO HEAL

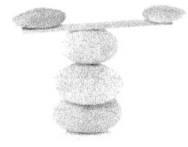

Exploring the Dimensions of Balance

Physical Balance: Physical balance is about keeping your body healthy through exercise, enough sleep, and eating right. It means moving your body regularly, getting the rest it needs to recover, and choosing foods that give it the right kind of fuel. It's about doing what's good for your body to keep it strong and working well. Organizations like the American Heart Association (AHA), the National Institute on Health (NIH), and others set guidelines and recommendations that can give you a base-point of what to follow to promote overall good health and wellness in addition to checking with your healthcare provider.

How do your physical health and activities contribute to your overall sense of balance?

Emotional Balance: Emotional balance is about managing your feelings in a way that sustains mental stability. It is recognizing your emotions, understanding them, and not letting them control your actions. Techniques like deep breathing, talking to friends, or taking time for hobbies, and helping others can help keep your emotions in check.

Recognizing and addressing emotional imbalances is important, as emotional well-being significantly contributes to a sense of fulfillment in life.

Reflect on how you manage emotions and stress. What practices help you maintain emotional equilibrium?

Professional and Personal Balance: Professional and personal balance is about dividing your time and energy in a way that works best for you and minimizes stress and unhealthy coping mechanisms. It means setting boundaries at work so you have time for family, friends, and activities you enjoy, ensuring neither side overwhelms the other. Achieving balance here is key to feeling fulfilled, as it allows space for both career achievements and personal happiness.

Imbalance in professional and personal balance can occur when you do not prioritize. Working excessively, overlooking personal time and relationships under the assumption that it's the right thing to do has its consequences. This can lead to burnout, a loss of enjoyment in life, and a spiral into strained relationships and dissatisfaction in other areas.

How do you navigate the demands of your professional life while fulfilling personal desires and responsibilities?

The Myths of Balance

Perfection Myth: Balance means that I must be perfect.

Reality: Balance does not mean perfection. Balance is not perfect.

Reflect on instances where the pursuit of perfection might have disrupted your sense of balance.

Productivity Myth: You are not successful unless you are busy.

Reality: Being busy doesn't always equate to being balanced, successful, or fulfilled.

How does your current level of busyness contribute to or distract you from your sense of balance?

Recognizing Signs of Imbalance

- Constant Fatigue
  Feeling tired all the time, regardless of rest.
- Irritability
  Small annoyances cause significant irritation.
- Sleep Issues
  Difficulty falling or staying asleep.
- Physical Symptoms
  Headaches, stomach issues, or other unexplained physical symptoms.
- Neglecting Personal Care
  Skipping meals, exercise, or hygiene routines.
- Withdrawal
  Pulling away from friends, family, or activities you once enjoyed.
- Overeating or Undereating
  Significant changes in eating habits.
- Lack of Concentration
  Difficulty focusing on tasks at work or home.
- Mood Swings
  Rapid changes in mood without a clear reason.
- Anxiety
  Persistent feelings of worry or unease.
- Depression

Feelings of sadness, hopelessness, or loss of interest in life.

- Substance Abuse

  Increasing reliance on alcohol, drugs, or medications.

- Work Obsession

  Thinking about work all the time, even during off hours.

- Neglecting Relationships

  Ignoring the needs of family and friends.

- Lack of Enjoyment

  Activities you once loved no longer bring pleasure.

- Perfectionism

  Striving for flawlessness and setting unreasonably high standards.

- Guilt Over Rest

  Feeling guilty for taking time to relax or do nothing.

- Procrastination

  Delaying or avoiding tasks, leading to stress.

- Burnout

  Feeling emotionally, mentally, and physically exhausted by your responsibilities.

- Negative Self Talk

  Undermining your own confidence with your words and impeding your ability to face life's challenges effectively.

- Feeling Unfulfilled

  Despite achievements, there's a sense of emptiness or lack of satisfaction.

Coping Mechanisms for Professional Women

Imbalanced Strategies

- Overcommitting
  Saying "yes" to every request or opportunity, leading to exhaustion and stress.
- Neglecting Self-Care
  Skipping meals, exercise, or rest for work.
- Isolation
  Reducing social and family interactions due to work commitments.
- Emotional Suppression
  Ignoring feelings of stress, frustration, or burnout.
- Work-Life Blur
  Allowing work to invade personal and family time.
- Impulsive Behaviors
  Resorting to shopping, binge-eating, or other quick fixes for stress relief.
- Avoidance
  Ignoring personal or family issues hoping they'll resolve on their own.
- Perfectionism
  Striving for flawless performance at work and home, creating unrealistic expectations.
- Digital Escapism
  Excessive use of social media or streaming to unwind.
- Physical Neglect
  Ignoring signs of physical weariness or health issues.

Balanced Strategies

- Setting Boundaries

  Knowing when to say "no" to protect time for self and family.

- Scheduled Self-Care

  Prioritizing regular meals, exercise, and rest.

- Quality Family Time

  Designating uninterrupted time for family activities and bonding.

- Emotional Awareness

  Recognizing and addressing feelings of stress or dissatisfaction.

- Defined Work Hours

  Establishing clear start and end times for work.

- Mindful Relaxation

  Engaging in meditation, reading, or other calming activities.

- Active Problem-Solving

  Addressing personal and family issues directly and constructively.

- Realistic Goals

  Setting achievable work and personal life goals.

- Digital Detox

  Limiting screen time to foster real-life connections.

- Positive Affirmations

  Focusing on positive words with a positive mindset

- Health Prioritization

  Regular health check-ups and attention to physical well-being.

Final Thoughts

Learning to have balance takes practice. Begin by tracking how you spend your time weekly. Categorize your activities and relationships into "Must Do," "Should Do," and "Nice to Do." Take time to consider the challenges or barriers of maintaining balance in today's fast-paced world. Be intentional and make time for balance. At the end of each week, reflect on whether your time allocation aligns with your priorities. What changes might you need to make to achieve a better balance? Write the changes. Make the changes and pivot when needed!

CHAPTER 2

LIGHT SHINES

It is safe to assume that the goal of all women is to provide a meaningful quality of life for their families. Yet, at what cost does this occur?

Whether your family consists of a child, pet, spouse, family member, or anyone else, in some way you are or will be a caregiver who provides for someone else. With that in mind, achieving your goal of caring for others always entails sacrifice. Often, we want other people to care about how and in what ways we sacrifice. We often want people to care in the way that we want them to care but that does not always occur.

> *You cannot have a logical conversation (about you) with people who do not care <u>about you</u> or the things that are important to you.*
>
> *Dr. Katherine Y. Brown*

It sounds very simple, but it's not. There comes a point in your life where you have to move on and work on healing yourself. Avoid seeking approval from others. The first approval must always come from you. So have you ever found yourself seeking praise, positive feedback, or validation from people who do not have your best intentions?

It's Time To Care About Yourself

Not everyone cares about you. There may be people in your life who want to see you fail. It's up to you to not fail. Don't let people who do not have your best interest win by giving up on your mental and physical health, your dreams or by failing. Re-shape your thinking and view failures as opportunities for growth and learning so that you keep getting back up, trying again, and progressing toward your goals. Not everyone has your best interest at heart.

Be careful who you share your thoughts, ideas, and emotions with. Have you ever asked a negative person for their feedback and as you expected, the response was negative? That's the point. In a need to find support from others, the greatest support system which resides within us is often overlooked.

Don't let people dim your light;
you have a purpose and you were meant to shine.

Did you know that you are amazing just the way that you are? Did you know that when you withhold your gifts and talents or allow your energy to be diverted toward things that aren't in line with your life's purpose, the world misses out on the talents you were meant to share? This discussion can take on various forms and dimensions.

Let's engage in dialogue with a few foundational questions.

Please don't rush through these questions as if they're only words on a page. Use the space below to write, journal, and respond to each question.

What is **your** purpose or assignment?

_____

_____

_____

_____

_____

_____

_____

_____

_____

_____

_____

_____

_____

_____

What are **you** doing?

_____

_____

_____

_____

_____

_____

_____

_____

We all have a purpose. What would **you** be doing if money was not a factor?

_____

_____

_____

_____

_____

_____

_____

_____

_____

Close your eyes and imagine a day when you're doing only what you love and what you are great at. What are you doing? What does a day in your life look like?

_____

_____

_____

_____

_____

_____

_____

_____

_____

_____

Final Thoughts

Your light is needed in this world. There is a missing piece in the universe that can only be fulfilled by you. You have a purpose. Embrace who you are with courage and honesty knowing that your worth isn't determined by external validation. The most important approval and validation happens within.

CHAPTER 3

CHERISHED MOMENTS

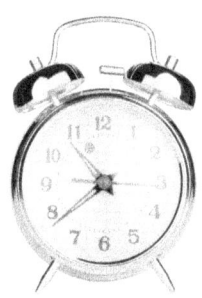

There are twenty-four hours in a day. We can't change yesterday because it's gone, and tomorrow is not here yet. So, how do we get our tasks done and keep everything balanced? Many find this hard, often feeling out of step or overwhelmed, and a big reason is that they aren't walking in their true purpose.

But here's a truth we often overlook: every choice we make involves sacrifice. When you're not walking in your purpose, you're not just losing out on achieving your dreams. You're sacrificing your unique talents and precious time, devoting them to someone else's vision, dreams, and aspirations.

Think about it. If you decide to follow your true calling, living out your unique purpose, what are you ready to sacrifice and give up? What are you willing to let go to fully live the life meant for you?

Conversely, when you drift on a path that isn't truly yours, you're giving up more than you may realize. You're letting go of your dreams, giving your time and skills to bring someone else's vision to life. Is that a sacrifice you're comfortable with?

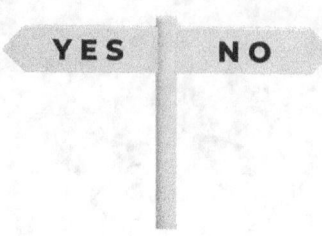

Every moment, and every choice has a cost. And every day you're not aligned with your purpose is a day spent paying a price. So, which costs are you willing to bear for the life you want?

What about the external indicators of success and fulfill- ment?

Just because you have awards, accolades, and honors does not mean that you have balance or that you are walking in your purpose. Isn't it interesting that we frequently look up to and admire women who we later find out are overwhelmed? We tend to confer awards based on extensive service and work records, but what about awards recognizing those who have an amazing quality of life?

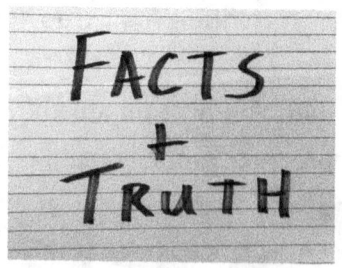

What would the world be like if conversations involved the truth when people asked us how we were doing?

What would life be like if we could feel **safe** responding with this?

"Right now, things are overwhelming. I joined a lot of organizations and neglected my husband and children. I now realize that I must have priorities. It's been difficult for me to get used to doing nothing in external organizations but I am learning each day that doing nothing with them allows me to do something with the people who matter most to me—my family."

Do you ask authentic questions?

_____

_____

_____

_____

_____

_____

Do you feel safe giving authentic and honest responses about how you are doing in life?

_____

_____

_____

_____

_____

_____

Maybe you are a new mother. Would you feel **safe** saying this?:

"Right now, things are difficult. I only wanted one child, but we have been blessed with three. I love being a wife and a mother, but on most days, I don't know who I am anymore. It's like my identity is slipping away. I began experiencing depression and sought counseling. I realized that there was nothing wrong with taking care of my mental and physical health. Depression is a real battle, and I nearly lost myself to overwhelming emotions. My husband and I now have someone watch the children one night a week so we can have a date night. I have also started doing things with the children that bring me joy. Life is getting better, one day at a time."

Write a statement you wish you could feel **safe** saying but do not say for fear of judgment.

_____

_____

_____

_____

_____

_____

All too often we are going through similar circumstances but because we hide behind our images and false perceptions of reality, we seldom realize that we are not alone in our experiences.

It's time that you own your story

- Love yourself from within.
- You deserve love, peace, joy, happiness, and **balance**.

The journey to balance requires us to be safe. For the remainder of this book, we will address several areas under the acronym: S.A.F.E. I created this acronym as a quick self check-in to respond to situations that challenge balance in life. When left unaddressed this may subsequently lead to imbalance.

S: Start with balance

- What are you balancing?

A: Assess how you define success

- How do you view internal success versus external success?

F: Find yourself through self-analysis

- What is the impact of your daily routine?

E: Explore goals and establish accountability

- What specific goals do you want to achieve, and how will you hold yourself accountable to them?

These four key areas form the word SAFE because when you are in sync with yourself, you generally are in a **SAFE** place.

Final Thoughts

The choices you make shape not only your days but your very essence. Embracing the S.A.F.E. approach isn't just about finding balance; it's about rediscovering and honoring yourself.

You must start each day with the intention to balance what truly matters. Assess your definition of success and ensure it resonates with your inner truth. Find yourself through self-analysis; understand the profound impact your daily routines have on your life. And finally, explore and establish goals with accountability, for they are the roadmap to your desired destination.

Remember, you're not alone in your experiences. Owning your truth, your story and sharing it authentically can be a powerful catalyst for change, not just for you but also for those around you who may be silently struggling with similar challenges. In life, strive to be in a place where you are S.A.F.E. - balanced, content, and aligned with your purpose.

Even when it does not feel like you are in control, you are in control. You have the power to create the life you desire and deserve. It's time to step forward with courage, embrace your journey, and shine in your unique light. Your story matters, and it's time that you own it with love and bravery.

CHAPTER 4

DEFINING BALANCE

Please know that I don't take lightly that you're still with me, turning the pages of this book. It's time for us to get to work. Think of this book as a journal and road map. Write in it, jot down notes and ideas, and embrace your journey. We'll start with balance.

Many women have allowed their overfilled day planners, agendas, and calendars to define success. This imbalance is perceived as successful by many. What is disturbing is that when we describe schedules that are not overbooked, we may not be perceived as successful.

Imbalance occurs when fulfillment is found based on how we are perceived by others.

Balance occurs when you identify and pursue what fulfills YOU not what fulfills others.

Learning what fulfills you may require you to unlearn what fulfillment looks like. Society, traditions, family, cultural norms, and other external variables contribute to what you perceive as balance or imbalance.

What fulfills you? Achieving balance when you are imbalanced must first start within you.

Meet Sally. She is a wife, a mother, doctoral-prepared, and a community leader.

Sally underwent a major life transition. Her marriage was in turmoil, despite her success as a prominent community figure. She had sacrificed so much for her achievements that she found herself in a dire financial position, struggling to cover her daily living expenses for food and shelter. Sally had invested countless hours in community service and networking with influential women in the community, including business owners, corporate executives, and high-profile elected officials. She regarded many of these women as not only mentors but also friends, as she had dedicated substantial time to meetings, late-night calls, and con-sistently answering their requests with a resounding "yes." Naturally, she believed these women were her support system and people she could trust.

However, when Sally mentioned her inability to pay her membership dues to organizations in which she held leadership positions, she was met with a disheartening response: "Maybe you should reconsider if you are the right fit to be a member. All members should be able to afford the dues, and if you can't, per-haps membership isn't suitable for you." She felt heartbroken and disillusioned that her mere disclosure of life challenges re-sulted in isolation from the group. Sally approached members individually and did not explicitly request financial assistance. Instead, she sought feedback, suggestions, and, in some cases, connections with fellow business leaders. Regrettably, her at-tempts yielded no positive response, and the reactions were so cold that she described them as piercing her heart. As a conse-quence, certain aspects of her marriage became strained due to the countless hours she dedicated to the community. Now, those with whom she had served turned their backs on her. In some ways, she had prioritized serving others over self-care, which led to an imbalance in her personal life. When her personal life became imbalanced, she found herself unable to turn to the circles where she had invested the majority of her time for any form of support. Feeling lost between two imbalanced worlds, unwanted by either, was an incredibly isolating position to be in.

When you are having personal challenges, it's good practice to develop a support system rather than share every challenge with anyone who will listen. Some will use your challenge as an opportunity to treat you less than the wonderful person that you are. I'm sure this may have happened to you in some aspect of your life albeit work, finances, marriage, relationships, etc.

There is a difference between a colleague and a confidant. What is the difference for you? What are the pros and cons of having each?

_____

_____

_____

_____

_____

_____

_____

_____

_____

_____

What can you learn from Sally's experience that you can apply to your life?

_____

_____

_____

_____

_____

_____

_____

_____

_____

_____

_____

_____

_____

_____

_____

_____

_____

_____

_____

Final Thoughts

Your journey to balance is personal and uniquely yours. It's not dictated by packed schedules or societal accolades but by a true sense of fulfillment and inner peace . What do you feel inside? Like Sally, many of us have found ourselves at the crossroads of external expectations and personal well-being. There is a fine line between being a dedicated individual and losing oneself in the pursuit of external validation.

The most significant measure of your success is how aligned you feel with your true self and purpose.

Consider carefully who you trust as confidants and how you cultivate your support system. Not everyone deserves a front-row seat in the story of your life. Cherish those who uplift you, understand the difference between colleagues and true supporters, and continue to embrace your path with wisdom and courage.

Your story is important, your dreams are valid, and your pursuit of balance is a testament to your strength and commitment to living a life filled with purpose and joy. Keep turning the pages of your life with intention, knowing that each chapter you write is a step closer to the truest version of yourself.

CHAPTER 5:
BALANCING ACT

We hear people use the term "balancing act" in various aspects of our lives. This may look different for each person depending on societal roles and responsibilities. What is the current state of balancing acts impacting women across our nation? We have come to a place where so-called "successful" women are burning the candle at both ends and not knowing which lighted path to follow. When we reflect on our lives and grasp how fleeting life is, it is important to determine if the paths pursued shall end in something meaningful, or end with having achieved nothing at all? Each path has an end destination.

Decisions, outcomes, and balancing priorities require momentum toward a goal. As we ascended to what is perceived as success, did our balancing acts keep us on the lighted path or did we find ourselves in an upside-down state of existence, spiraling out of control, nearing disaster in various aspects of life—whether physical, financial, emotional, or spiritual?

Balancing family, companions, work, and personal needs are all essential for self-preservation. Yet, with many priorities competing for your attention, it is important to contemplate and make a clear choice between attempting to tackle everything in a twenty-three-hour period, leaving just one hour for yourself, and slowing down to count the cost of each assignment with the aim of accomplishing things in accordance to your priorities.

Making Time For You

You may ask yourself, "How do I determine the things that fulfill my purpose, benefitting not just myself but also my family and children? How do I manage business while meeting my own needs? How can I regain something for myself after giving so much to others? How do I prevent giving away all of myself? Have I reached a point where I've given so much of myself that I no longer recognize who I am? When do I choose to have fun with the family or focus on having fun for myself and by myself?"

If your heart is racing, your hands are shaking, and you're spiraling out of control but the image you have created of yourself in society does not allow you to seek help, it's time to find balance. You're reading the right book. I am proud of you for taking the time, right now, to focus on yourself. Stay focused. Keep reading. You can do this.

Race, age, creed, nor color are factors in this journey. Whether you're married, engaged, single, widowed, or in a life partnership is not relevant to this journey. The only factors are those that yield answers to the following questions. Take a few moments to pause, reflect, then answer these questions.

Who are you?

_____

_____

_____

_____

_____

_____

Who have you become?

_____

_____

_____

_____

_____

_____

Who are you becoming?

_____

_____

_____

_____

_____

_____

Do you like the person in your mirror?

_____

_____

_____

_____

_____

_____

_____

Who does she serve?

_____

_____

_____

_____

_____

_____

What brings you joy?

_____

_____

_____

_____

_____

_____

_____

These may be difficult questions, and your heart may be burdened by feelings of hurt, confusion, anger, or even numbness. Perhaps you are experiencing none of these emotions. Regardless of your current state, go back, take time and make an effort to thoughtfully answer these questions. This will become part of your foundation for growth.

Define Yourself On Your Own Terms

Define yourself on your own terms, provide details, be honest, and put it down on paper. Remember, where you are now doesn't have to be your final destination. Self-reflection can be a part of your journey if you fully embrace the process. Don't rush it; allow it to unfold naturally.

Pause.

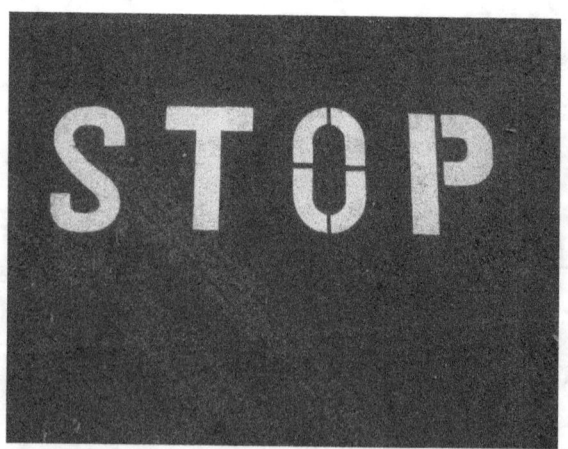

Now that we have reflected on several very important questions, ask yourself, What have you learned?

_____

_____

_____

_____

_____

_____

_____

_____

_____

_____

Please, do not rush to the next page of this book until you pause, reflect, and take a personal inventory of the questions that you have just been asked. Write the first words or thoughts that come to your mind. Take a few days if needed.

_____

_____

_____

_____

_____

_____

_____

_____

_____

_____

Final Thoughts

Realizing that there is a choice between balance and imbalance is critical. The journey to balance doesn't mean that there will always be perfect equilibrium. Life will happen, but you are in control of your response, your actions, and bringing harmony to your life. The questions posed aren't just queries; they are guiding you toward deeper self-awareness and understanding.

This isn't about quick fixes or easy answers. It's about honoring your truth, recognizing your worth, and understanding that your balancing act is a personal dance that only you can choose. Embrace the uncertainty and the complexity of it all because this is where genuine growth happens.

As you continue balancing your balancing act, carry with you the knowledge that each step, each reflection, and each moment of honesty brings you closer to the life you're meant to live – one filled with purpose, joy, and balance. Your journey is significant, your experiences are valid, and your pursuit of balance requires your strength and resilience.

Keep turning these pages, keep reading, keep asking these questions, keep reflecting, and keep striving for a life that feels authentically yours. The path may be winding, but it's yours, and every step is a step toward the person you're meant to become. Be patient and trust your process.

CHAPTER 6:
FINDING SAFETY

There is a self-destructive aspect within each of us that we must confront and break free from. Perhaps yours manifest as overeating, overworking, neglecting relaxation, or even not allowing yourself to rest. Maybe your self-destructive side is concealed beneath low self-esteem or in another area that remains unseen by others.

Let's Consider A Holistic Approach To Self: We must deal with our emotional imbalance before it creates physical imbalance.

Does your pleasure come from within, or does it depend on external validation for your sense of fulfillment?

_____

_____

_____

_____

_____

_____

_____

Meet six women with whom you may have some commonality. You may know them, you may be them, or you may avoid them.

Ms. Backstabber

I'll stab you in the back so that I can shine in the eyes of others. I will offer to partner with you on your idea but when people say it's a good idea, I take charge, tell you that I don't need your help, and when I run out of ideas, I quickly let you know how you can assist me. I tell you that we can present the idea on Wednesday, but I have an ulterior agenda to present it on my own on Monday. I'm not trustworthy but if you mention it to me, I will become defensive and rally as many supporters as I can to support my agenda and me. Because I create successful circles around me, I often succeed. I'm really an attention seeker. I have a need to be liked and I will satisfy that need at any cost.

She is imbalanced and does not feel SAFE!

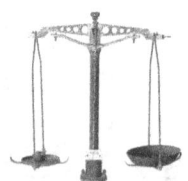

Women who hurt other women are also experiencing hurt in some other areas of their lives. Whether you are Ms. Backstabber or if you continue to allow yourself to be subjected to Ms. Backstabber it's time for a change.

Let's get SAFE!

S: Start with balance - What are you balancing?

A: Assess how you define success - How do you view internal success versus external success?

F: Find yourself through self-analysis - What is the impact of your daily routine?

E: Explore goals and establish accountability.

Ms. Please Like Me

I know right from wrong but I want to be known as a peace-maker, and I'm scared to step up and say what I believe in. I pretty much say yes to everything. For instance, I told the kids that I would take them to Fun World this weekend, but the president of an organization said they needed me to attend a meeting. I am intelligent, beautiful, and appear to have the perfect family. Many people want to be like me. I'm really stressed out, lonely, and overwhelmed with my situation. My day planner is so full that I can't enjoy "downtime" with my husband, children, or family. I fill my circle with people who admire me, but they don't know my true feelings because I would rather appear to be happy and perfect than express my true ideas and opinions.

She is imbalanced and does not feel SAFE!

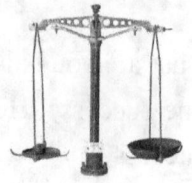

Let's get SAFE!

S: Start with Balance - What are you balancing?

A: Assess how you define Success - How do you view internal success versus external success?

F: Find yourself through self-analysis - What is the impact of your daily routine?

E: Explore goals and establish accountability.

Ms. Picture Perfect, Closet Promiscuous

I spend my day making others think that I have it all but at the end of the day, I really have nothing. Many of my friendships and relationships are primarily built on wealth, and I'm aware that if the money were to disappear, those relationships might fade too. I'm a single parent with two children. I have no problem being intimate with a married man or any man because I want to be loved. I'm really depressed and have low self-esteem. I'm beautiful but I don't know it. I'm strong, powerful, and intelligent but when I look in the mirror, I do not see any of this. A lot of people say I have everything together. I've learned to focus on what matters most and for me, that's doing whatever needs to be done to feel emotions from others.

She is imbalanced and does not feel SAFE!

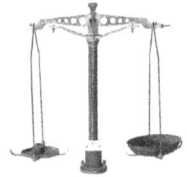

Let's get SAFE!

S: Start with balance - What are you balancing?

A: Assess how you define success - How do you view internal success versus external success?

F: Find yourself through self-analysis - What is the impact of your daily routine?

E: Explore goals and establish accountability.

Mrs. Happily Married with Children

I project an image that marriage is effortless, but the reality is that I did not realize how much time it takes to have a success-ful marriage. I neglect my spouse and family for meetings be-cause the roles of wife and mother are consuming. I was more focused on portraying the American dream of having children, a house, a car, and a husband and now I find that I feel lost, alone, and I don't know if I am really happy. I went from being a successful person who people admired to my role of mother and wife and I honestly don't know who I am anymore. No one told me that this would be easy, but I have isolated myself from being able to ask for help.

She is imbalanced and does not feel SAFE!

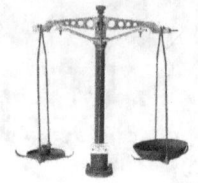

Let's get SAFE!

S: Start with balance - What are you balancing?

A: Assess how you define success - How do you view internal success versus external success?

F: Find yourself through self-analysis - What is the impact of your daily routine?

E: Explore goals and establish accountability.

Ms. I'm Happy To Be Divorced

My spouse and I had irreconcilable differences, which ultimately led to our divorce. Due to my spouse and I being highly visible in the community, everyone is aware of the divorce. While infidelity was one of the issues among others, looking back, I recognize that I didn't seek wise counsel when making the decision to divorce. I acted impulsively, driven by emotions and concerns about what others would think, especially since my husband's infidelity was not discreet. Consequently, I now feel insecure because it seems like "everyone" knows about it. Despite outwardly portraying happiness and even celebrating with an "I am divorced" party, I'm secretly miserable. My spouse and I still conduct business together because we have many financial ties. The truth is, if I hadn't been so concerned about how others perceived me, I would have sought marriage counseling, wise counsel, spiritual guidance, and professional help before letting my emotions dictate my actions. In my view, we might still be married. I am a successful businesswoman in the community, with a home, car, wardrobe, and thriving business that attest to my success. However, on the inside, I'm grappling with aging, loneliness, and a growing sense of being lost. I wonder if I will ever find love again.

She is imbalanced and does not feel SAFE!

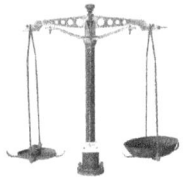

Let's get SAFE!

S: Start with Balance - What are you balancing?

A: Assess how you define Success - How do you view internal success versus external success?

F: Find yourself through Self Analysis - What is the impact of your daily routine?

E: Explore Goals and establish accountability.

Ms. I Don't Remember Who She Is

I have spent years being everything to everyone. I smile and laugh on cue. I understand how to navigate political circles. I know what clothing to wear to stand out in the crowd. I have been hurt by many organizations but I know how to navigate and rise to success. In intimate settings when titles don't matter, I am uncomfortable; in fact, I am an introvert. I do not know how to engage with people when it is not focused on a goal. Most, if not all of my relationships are based on someone wanting something. I have gotten older and am in the top leadership positions of my organizations but for some reason, I now realize that my circle is composed of people who are not my true friends. I have spent time and over fifty years in elite organizations with other women of influence and now suddenly I feel lost. I have a difficult time identifying fact from fiction in others and in myself. I don't know who I am anymore. I am very confused because I created myself around who others wanted me to be. My memory is not as sharp as it used to be and I don't remember where I began, where I ended, or what has happened to me. I am in distress. It is time for me to reinvent myself but I don't know who that self should be.

She is imbalanced and does not feel SAFE!

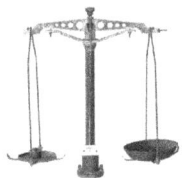

Let's get SAFE!

S: Start with Balance - What are you balancing?
A: Assess how you define Success - How do you view internal success versus external success?
F: Find yourself through Self Analysis - What is the impact of your daily routine?
E: Explore Goals and establish accountability.

The stories of these women and how they use the safe acronym are examples to help demonstrate behavioral change in life. Each decision you make, each challenge you face, and each moment of introspection is about personal growth, taking control, and enjoying peace in your own life. Learning, and having the courage to take responsibility for your choice is powerful on the road to balance.

Having traveled nationwide and interviewed numerous women, I can assure you that the stories shared here represent just a glimpse of the experiences women have reported. The key message is straightforward: your true and authentic self should be the only self you embrace. When we deviate from our authentic selves, it can lead to emotional imbalances, which can eventually manifest as physical imbalances that may jeopardize our integrity, happiness, and overall well-being.

You may still be asking yourself, why did I take the time to introduce you to those women? Let me elaborate. Here's the reality: we all have a story. We all navigate through personal complexities in different ways.

We all have something that we are unhappy with or have been unhappy with that we portray to others as being amazingly well. Whether you choose to share these intimate thoughts with others or not, after speaking with thousands of women over the years, I can assure you that there's no challenge you're going through that someone else hasn't experienced. There are numerous examples that could have been provided, but I'll leave it up to you to speak your own truth and determine what you need to feel SAFE.

Final Thoughts

Reflect on the stories of these women and recognize the common thread that binds all of our narratives together – the goal for authenticity and balance. Each story is a mirror, reflecting parts of our own lives, choices, and perhaps the faces we show to the world.

Understanding and embracing your true self isn't always easy or straightforward. The most profound balance you can achieve is not between the roles and responsibilities you juggle but the challenges within yourself. This is where imbalance can occur when you feel you are not enough, so you keep adding and adding until you lose yourself in commitments that may not align with your purpose. It's the perception of unfulfillment that occurs even though everything we have symbolizes a life that is fulfilled yet we are unhappy.

Take a moment and ask yourself, what does it mean to be

authentically you? How can you move closer to a life that feels genuinely balanced and fulfilling? These aren't just questions to ponder; they are requirements for the life you were meant to lead.

As you turn the page to the next chapter of this book and your life, carry with you the courage to face and embrace your true self. Let the stories of Ms. Backstabber, Ms. Please Like Me, and others serve not as warnings but as reminders that you must be in a place in life where you feel SAFE, balanced, and whole.

The journey to self-discovery and balance is ongoing; it's a dynamic process. Each day offers a new opportunity to align more closely with the person you're meant to be. Embrace it with an open heart and mind. You always have a choice, and there will always be a consequence for your actions. Make sure you are okay with the decisions you make.

CHAPTER 7:
COMPETING PRIORITIES

Generally, women balance several things at one time. We are amazing and talented at multitasking. The balancing act is three-tiered: family, business/work, and personal/self. Family may encompass caring for aging parents, siblings, relatives, spouses, or children. Business and work in your life may involve professional responsibilities, that include employment and your involvement with organizations in the community or church. Personal needs and self should always be the priority, yet with many competing priorities they can be mistakenly left void.

Keeping the balls in the air

Imagine a juggler who keeps balancing balls in the air. What are you balancing? Are you like a juggler with plates that are about to fall? To master the balancing act you must:

1. Take care of your physical, mental, and emotional health;

2. Identify what you need to do to recharge your battery for the next day;

3. Realize that often we think we are recharging our batteries but in reality, we are not using our time effectively;

4. Take a daily appraisal to determine how much effective time you are using to rejuvenate yourself.

Before we proceed, respond to the following questions:

1. How do you take care of your physical, mental, and emotional health? Be specific. Include when and how.

_____

_____

_____

_____

_____

_____

_____

_____

_____

2. What three things do you do to recharge your battery (mental and physical health) in life for the day ahead? Be specific. After you write these, reflect and make sure these are things you actually did in the last thirty days.

_____

_____

_____

_____

_____

_____

_____

_____

_____

_____

_____

3. What outcomes in your life usually let you know that you have recharged your batteries? Be specific.

_____

_____

_____

_____

_____

_____

_____

_____

_____

_____

4. What are three ways that you are successful at taking care of yourself? Be specific.

_____

_____

_____

_____

_____

_____

_____

_____

_____

_____

Based on what you wrote above, if you don't feel you are successful in these areas, write where you are today and where you hope to be in the 30-60-90 days. This is a work in progress.

Final Thoughts

Balance in your life is something you actively create each day. It's about making choices that fit your life and needs. Taking care of yourself isn't just one more task on your to-do list; it's the foundation of everything you do. Always consider the ways you care for your body and mind, and how you recharge. This isn't about perfection. It's about making small, consistent changes that add up over time. Keep asking yourself what works for you and what doesn't. You can change your mind unapologetically when things, situations, and people no longer work for your balance. This is your life, and you have the power to shape it in a way that feels right for you.

CHAPTER 8:
FINDING FULFILLMENT

Success is all in your perception. How do you view success? Take at least three quiet minutes with your eyes closed and answer the question: What does success look like? START NOW! Don't proceed with reading until you do this.

SERIOUSLY! STOP READING AND ANSWER THE QUESTION!!!

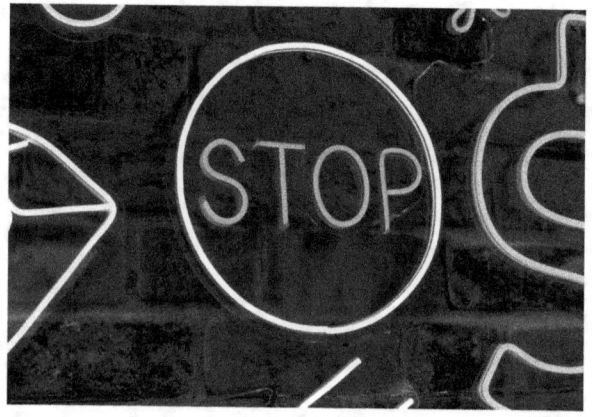

Welcome back.

Now that you have that image in your mind, let's proceed. Why did I have you capture that image in your mind? There is something or someone that you observed who shaped your image of what success looks like. Who is that person? Starting here is important because this individual or image is likely a benchmark against which you measure yourself and your achievements.

What about this person led you to believe they were successful?

Write it.

Write everything that comes to mind from the mental picture you have of them.

_____

_____

_____

_____

_____

_____

_____

_____

_____

Were they overworked?

_____

_____

_____

_____

_____

_____

_____

_____

_____

How do you know?

_____

_____

_____

_____

_____

_____

_____

_____

_____

_____

Did they tell you or did you observe it?

_____

_____

_____

_____

_____

_____

_____

_____

_____

_____

_____

What did you observe?

_____

_____

_____

_____

_____

_____

_____

_____

_____

_____

What would those closest to them say about their success?

_____

_____

_____

_____

_____

_____

_____

_____

_____

_____

_____

Explore deeper. What would these people say about their success?

Children?

_____

_____

_____

_____

_____

_____

_____

_____

Spouse?

_____

_____

_____

_____

_____

_____

_____

_____

_____

Family/Friends?

_____

_____

_____

_____

_____

_____

_____

_____

_____

Co-workers?

_____

_____

_____

_____

_____

_____

_____

_____

_____

_____

_____

Employer?

_____

_____

_____

_____

_____

_____

_____

_____

_____

If these individuals have children, would their children share memories of enjoying their mother, or would they recount stories of a mother who was often distracted and too preoccupied for school plays, too exhausted to read a book at night? It's common for us to assess people based on their possessions without looking beneath the surface to understand who they truly are.

Would they be described as a person who instead of helping with homework, spent evenings attending meetings followed by calls to colleagues to vent about their meeting frustrations? Sometimes, we base our reality on others and then realize that what we thought we wanted was not really good for us or that it did not make us happy.

External happiness is one of the worst indicators of success. The car, house, wardrobe, shoes, dog, polished-to-perfection look, awards, bank account, or the appearance of the bank account may say success but...

Are you happy?

You must assess how you define success. How do you view internal success versus external success?

Success: External Happiness

External happiness often gets measured by materialistic achievements and societal benchmarks. It's the job title you hold, the car you drive, the house you live in, and the clothes you wear. It's quantifiable, visible to others, and often, what's expected by society. But it can leave you chasing an endless cycle of "more" without ever feeling truly fulfilled.

Success: Internal Happiness

Internal happiness, on the other hand, is deeply personal and less tangible. It's about feeling content, fulfilled, and at peace with your life and choices, regardless of external circumstances. It involves understanding your values, aligning your actions with your beliefs, and finding joy in the journey rather than just the destination. It's not something that can be compared or measured against others but is about how you feel about yourself and your life.

Your Perception is Your Reality

Your perception is your reality and the choice is yours. No matter what you choose, if you don't feel balanced inside, it will eventually lead to imbalance. The reality you perceive and live by is often a reflection of your inner state and choices. Recognizing this power is the first step towards seeking a life that is truly fulfilling and balanced. The choice is yours.

Final Thoughts

Keep thinking about what success really means to you. It's easy to get caught up in what everyone else sees as success, but what matters most is how you feel about your own life and achievements. Real success isn't just about what you have or what you've done. It's about being true to yourself and finding happiness in your own way. Keep this in mind as you move forward, and don't be afraid to redefine success on your own terms. You can change your view of success and find balance in a world of imbalance. Your life is yours to live, and you're the one who decides what makes it successful.

CHAPTER 9

EMBRACING CHANGE

The challenge that many women face is that they often don't look beyond the invisible veil of success—the facade that conceals their real issues. Consequently, they develop false perceptions of who people truly are. Many women spend their lives making sacrifices in an attempt to become like someone they perceive as successful when the unfortunate truth is that the person they aspire to be is actually miserable. Ultimately, the person in your mirror determines whether you are successful or not successful. You can be bank-account rich and happiness poor.

My favorite holiday memory was when my mother wasn't working. We used aluminum foil and newspaper comic strips as wrapping paper, free clothing gift boxes from the store, and baked cookies that we filled each box with as Christmas gifts. My mother was generally one to work long hours and what she didn't realize was that, as an only child, what I valued most was that time with her. That's all most children and families ever want: uninterrupted time together.

Do you give your family your time? It doesn't matter how you define your family. It could be a pet, spouse, children, parent, sibling, etc. You can also have chosen family, the people around you that matter most.

Once you identify your definition of family. Now, reflect on whether you dedicate enough of your time to your family.

_____

_____

_____

_____

_____

_____

_____

_____

Being present means that you must be attentive and engaged in the moment. Time is not the same as quality time. Are you spending quality time with your family?

Are you engaged with each other in dialogue or do you define family time as everyone being in the same room while preoccupied with something else?

_____

_____

_____

_____

_____

_____

_____

_____

How do you enjoy each other's company? Be specific.

_____

_____

_____

_____

_____

_____

_____

_____

_____

_____

Is it a challenge to give your family uninterrupted time with you? If so, explain why.

_____

_____

_____

_____

_____

_____

_____

_____

_____

_____

What does being present look like to you? Explain the observable behaviors.

_____

_____

_____

_____

_____

_____

_____

_____

Your presence does not matter if you are not engaged and present.

At a music performance that had concluded, one of the performers asked me if I had seen their mother. I complimented them on their performance and then directed them to where I had seen their parents. To my surprise, when they thanked me for the compliment they additionally remarked, "At least you saw the performance. My mother was on her cell phone working the entire time. I looked at her almost the entire time and she never looked back at me because she was on her phone."

Are you embracing the moments in life or preparing to share the moments via social media to create a picture of your life the way that you want others to view you? *Take time to participate in the life moments that matter most.*

Final Thoughts

It's easy to get caught up in the race for what looks good on the outside, but remember, real contentment comes from what's happening inside of you. Think about what true success and happiness mean to you. **The most valuable asset you have is your time.** You can spend money and eventually get it back, but when you give your time, that is a gift that can never be returned, replaced, or redeemed. Time that has passed is gone forever. How you spend your time, especially with those you care about, reflects your priorities and values. Don't let the lure of a seemingly perfect life on social media or in other places you observe dictate how you live your own life. Be present, truly present, in the moments that matter. This isn't about grand gestures but the small, everyday actions that show love and care.

Keep asking yourself if you're living the life you want or one that's expected of you. This is a tough question, and sometimes you have to ask it more than once because societal expectations may be deeply ingrained in your routine. It's okay if this has happened; it is not too late. Your path to balance and fulfillment is yours to shape. Make sure it aligns with your values and brings you joy. Your life was never meant to be just a series of tasks to be completed. Life is a gift to you; it's yours, so cherish it.

CHAPTER 10:
MENTAL DETOX

There is a need for honesty and transparency among women. Ask yourself: Do you desire to be loved for who you truly are, or for a facade? Creating one false image inevitably leads to more, perpetuating a cycle of insincerity. Remember, if people dislike the real you, perhaps they aren't the right company for your journey. It's essential, at times, to focus more on loving yourself and less on seeking validation from those who don't genuinely support your success. Being busy doesn't necessarily equate to being productive.

Prioritize what truly matters.

To prioritize means to give your full attention to things that matter most to you in a specific order. In life there will always be something that pulls on you for attention. However, since you cannot clone yourself, you have to be disciplined with how you spend your time. This means that some things are just more important than others. Identify what brings you joy and pursue it.

What is success and happiness if you can't enjoy it?

Are you productive with your family, work, and time set aside for yourself, in all aspects of your life with no loopholes or regret?

_____

_____

_____

_____

_____

_____

_____

_____

_____

Introduction to the 30-Day Commitment

Today is a great day for you to commit to making yourself happier. This may sound easier said than done, but I encourage you to make a thirty-day commitment to yourself. Do one thing each day that will help to make you a better YOU. Add your own questions and comments once you finish this list.

It's commonly said that it takes thirty days to form a habit. I want you to use the next thirty days to cultivate a habit of loving yourself. What's on the inside will eventually radiate outward. Your internal self is crucial, and the perception of unfulfillment is often rooted in external factors. Therefore, let go of the "what if," "should be," and "could have been," and focus on you. You may accomplish this self work by intentionally doing the following:

Day 1: Begin the day by watching the sunrise in silence. Let gratitude be at the center of your thoughts and focus. Allow yourself to be rooted in gratitude and what that means for you in your life.

Day 2: Watch the sunset in silence. Say the word 'smile' and focus on happiness.

Day 3: Do not participate in any form of gossip at work, at home, with family, friends, walk away from gossip.

Day 4: Send a "thank you" or a "thinking-of-you" card to someone who helped you at least ten years ago.

Day 5: Make a quiet dinner for you and a family member.

Day 6: Go for a walk outside.

Day 7: Take a break from all social media that is not work-related.

Day 8: Practice meditation for thirty minutes.

Day 9: Take a free yoga class. You can often find free ones in parks, at community centers, or even online.

Day 10: Volunteer your time. For example, you can volunteer at an animal shelter for the day.

Day 11: Say "no" to any outside commitments that you are not required to participate in.

Day 12: Take a one day class that explores the arts. This can be quilting, sewing, candle making or some other class that incorporates the arts.

Day 13: Identify free events happening in your community. Take time to explore the exhibits, museums, and free resources.

Day 14: Listen and watch the birds outside. Do not talk on your phone. Sit in silence and enjoy nature for at least sixty minutes.

Day 15: Write a list of at least twenty specific things that you are grateful for.

Day 16: Go to a movie theater or a play by yourself and enjoy the show.

Day 17: Have a staycation in your home. Appreciate the things that you have been blessed with.

Day 18: Turn on a fun song and dance for at least ten minutes.

Day 19: Identify a positive quote or affirmation that inspires you and program your phone to alert you every three hours with that quote or affirmation. Read it out loud when the alert comes up.

Day 20: Call someone who makes you laugh. Enjoy the conversation.

Day 21: Eat! Go out to eat by yourself, treat yourself to a nutritious meal.

Day 22: Sleep. We often lack proper rest.Practice sleep hygiene to guarantee you get the amount of sleep that helps you to feel your best.

Day 23: Sometimes we have an abundance and we don't realize that there are other people in need. Clean your closet and donate at least one large bag of shoes, clothing, or other items.

Day 24: Buy five $5 dollar gift cards and give them to five strangers you meet throughout the day.

Day 25: If you go through a drive-thru restaurant, pay for the order of the car behind you.

Day 26: Look in the mirror and say at least ten positive things about yourself.

Day 27: Spend another day at the park. If you are physically able, get on the swing and two other pieces of playground equipment that you enjoyed as a child. Embrace your inner child.

Day 28: Identify one thing that you have never done and have the courage to do it today while alone in silence. Maybe it's taking a nature walk. Enjoy the process.

Day 29: Identify twenty accomplishments that you have that you are proud of. Yes, I said twenty. Don't overlook any step of your life's accomplishments. Only you can define accomplishment. Have peace in what you have accomplished; be happy with you. Remember, if you have been blessed with success once, you can be blessed again.

Day 30: Identify thirty amazing things that you will do for yourself for the next thirty days. Thirty is a lot, but you are worth it .

Reflection and Ongoing Practice

Notice that this list is not heavily involved with spending money; instead, it's about self-reflection and investing time in yourself. Your happiness is crucial. Feel free to revisit these activities whenever you need a boost. Always be aware of who you are and never create an image based on what you perceive in others or what you think others expect of you. Focus on creating a happy space for yourself. When you feel overwhelmed, slow down, focus on your breathing, visualize something positive, meditate, and ensure each day includes a moment of positivity.

Final Thoughts

Perception is your reality, and the choice is yours. No matter what path you choose, if you don't feel balanced internally, it will lead to external imbalance. Focus on nurturing your inner self, and watch as your world transforms. I encourage you to bookmark this chapter and revisit it often. Let it be a guiding post for you as you continue through this book and beyond. Revisiting these practices can help reaffirm your commitment to your happiness and balance. Remember, the journey to self-fulfillment is ongoing, and this chapter can serve as a valuable resource whenever you need to realign with your goals and aspirations. The choice, as always, is yours.

CHAPTER 11:
MENTORSHIP MATTERS

Contrary to what you may have led yourself to believe, we all have issues. It is not by chance that I keep reinforcing this statement. Regardless of how good you look, the brand of car you drive, ownership of a private jet, or how large your bank account is, we all have issues. So many women feel that their colleagues are perfect and that they themselves are the only flawed people in the world. This couldn't be farther from the truth. Unfortunately, as most people search to validate themselves, they often do not tell you the areas in their lives that they struggle with as well. This creates a false sense of reality and self. The desire to create a facade of happiness has subsequently led us to create an infectious cycle of mistrust that can continue running unrestrained.

What is a solution to this you may ask? Mentorship. There is a significant need to have honest and transparent mentors who are invested in helping other women succeed. When women feel like they are failures and alone with no one who can understand their concerns, imbalance occurs.

The real opportunities for mentorship among women have lessened. Either by virtue of the mentor with fear of being exceeded by the mentee, or by mentees who lack respect and values of appreciating the time and contributions that the mentor provides. Many women find that as we elevate up the ladder of success, we lose mentors.

As our bank accounts increase, we find ourselves "membership" rich and "confidant" poor. While someone may have many affiliations or connections, they often lack deep, intimate relationships with true confidants.

When the economy took a negative spiral, jobs were lost, finances were diminished, and there were women (married and single) who were in leadership positions in the most prestigious women's organizations who couldn't feed their families, yet their position in society placed them where they did not feel safe to seek assistance from others. It doesn't seem acceptable to have women give their time and talents to serve in groups with people, but when they are in need, they have nowhere to turn. This is why mentorship is important. The duration, frequency, location for mentorship should always be explored in collaboration.

Having a powerful mentor makes a difference. There are many types of mentors. Below are a few common ones.

- Traditional Mentorship: This involves a one-on-one relationship between a mentor and mentee, where the mentor provides guidance, knowledge, and advice to support the mentee's personal and professional growth. It's often characterized by a more experienced individual guiding someone less experienced.

- Peer Mentorship: In this model, individuals of similar professional levels or ages mentor each other. It's based on the premise that peers can offer valuable insights and support because they're likely facing similar challenges and can share recent experiences and solutions.

- Group Mentorship: This involves a single mentor or a group of mentors working with multiple mentees. It allows for a diverse range of perspectives and experiences to be shared, fostering a collaborative learning environment.

- Reverse Mentorship: This innovative approach flips the traditional mentor-mentee relationship, with the younger or less experienced individual serving as the mentor. It's particularly useful in areas like technology, social media, and current trends, where younger generations might have more expertise.

- Virtual Mentorship: Leveraging technology, virtual mentorship allows mentors and mentees to connect remotely via email, messaging platforms, video calls, and other digital means. It's flexible and accessible, making it ideal for global and diverse connections.

- Flash Mentorship: This is a short-term mentorship arrangement focused on specific, immediate goals or problems. It's akin to a "mentorship session" rather than an ongoing relationship, useful for targeted advice and quick guidance.

- Career Mentorship: Specifically focused on the mentee's professional development, this type involves guidance on career paths, job transitions, skill development, and networking within the industry.

- Life Mentorship: This broader and more holistic approach goes beyond professional advice to include guidance on personal development, work-life balance, and overall well-being.

Mentorship is empowering women, serving as a catalyst for both personal and professional growth. It offers a supportive framework where experienced mentors provide guidance, share invaluable insights, and facilitate networking opportunities, enabling mentees to navigate the complexities of their careers and personal development with confidence. For women, who often face unique challenges in the workplace and society, such as gender bias and limited access to leadership roles, mentorship can be especially transformative. It not only helps in building skills and knowledge but also boosts self-esteem and resilience, encouraging women to break through barriers, aspire for higher achievements, and support one another. This creates a ripple effect, fostering a culture of empowerment and equality that benefits not just the individuals involved but also the broader community.

Understanding Mentorship

Mentorship creates a dynamic relationship where a more experienced or knowledgeable individual supports and guides someone less experienced. This partnership is about nurturing growth, offering support, and providing insights that are crucial for overcoming complex challenges.

What Mentorship Is Not

Mentorship is not a one-sided interaction focused only on the mentor imparting wisdom. It's not about fostering dependency or imposing one's path onto another. This relationship isn't defined by superiority but by mutual respect and a shared commitment to growth. It's not about making decisions for another; rather, it's about learning to make informed choices through the guidance and experiences shared.

Identifying a Mentor and Setting Boundaries

Selecting a mentor involves identifying someone whose values resonate with yours and who has navigated the path you're embarking on. Respect, not just for their achievements but also for their wisdom and character, is paramount. They should demonstrate a genuine interest in your development and be willing to invest their time and energy into your progress.

Clearly defined boundaries and structure are vital for a successful mentorship. Discuss and agree upon how often and through which means (phone, in-person, video conference) you will meet. Determine the duration of each session and set a timeline for the mentorship's duration. This structure ensures both parties respect each other's time and commitments and provides a framework for consistent progress.

When seeking a mentor, be realistic in expectations. Determine what you want from the relationship; how often do you plan to communicate? Do not substitute an email for a handwritten card or offer to bring a cup of coffee or lunch to your meeting.

When serving as a mentor, be approachable, and set clear parameters. Be honest with the advice that you would have wanted someone else to share with you. In either case, there is no need to fear that the transference of knowledge from mentor to mentee is negative. Both can learn from the other. If what is meant for you is for you, there is no need to fear sharing knowledge with others.

Final Thoughts

Now that we have explored some of the pervasive issues of superficial success and the deep-seated need for genuine connection and guidance, take time to reflect on mentorship. This is a tool that has the capacity to nurture growth and understanding, offering hope in a world often overshadowed by competition and isolation.

As you consider the role mentors have played in your life and how they've helped shape your path, also think about stepping into this role yourself.

Becoming a mentor isn't just about passing on wisdom and experiences; it's about recognizing the right time and the right person. While there's always an opportunity to guide others, it's important to choose whom you mentor thoughtfully. Mentoring someone on the same platform as you might seem ideal, but it can inadvertently lead to competition due to the similarities in your journeys. Instead, there are times when it will be best to seek out those whose paths are different enough that your guidance becomes a bridge to new understandings rather than a mirror reflecting back your own challenges.

Remember, the road towards balance and fulfillment is continuous and ever-evolving. Seek out those who inspire and guide you, and be that source of inspiration for others when the time is right.

Always remember to be mindful of the dynamics at play in mentorship, and choose to mentor in situations where you can foster growth, not competition.

We can break the cycle of mistrust and build a future where every woman feels supported, valued, and empowered. By carefully choosing not only who mentors you but also who you decide to mentor, you ensure that the exchange enriches all lives involved. It also fosters growth, understanding, and a deeper sense of balance.

Sample Mentorship Checklists

For Mentees:

☑ **Define Your Goals:**
What do you want to achieve through mentorship?

☑ **Research Potential Mentors:**
Look for individuals whose career paths, skills, or experiences align with your goals.

☑ **Prepare to Reach Out:**
Draft an email, letter, or plan what you'll say during an initial meeting or phone call.

☑ **Set Initial Meeting:**
Discuss your goals, expectations, and what you hope to gain from the mentorship.

☑ **Discuss Availability:**

How often will you meet, and through what means (in-person, phone, video conference)?

☑ **Set Agendas for Meetings:**

Plan what you'll discuss or what advice you need in advance.

☑ **Reflect on Meetings:**

After each meeting, note what you learned and any follow-up actions you need to take.

☑ **Show Gratitude:**

Regularly express appreciation for your mentor's time and advice.

☑ **Evaluate Progress:**

Periodically assess what you've learned and how it's helping you towards your goals.

☑ **Provide Feedback:**

Share with your mentor how their guidance is impacting your goals.

For Mentors:

☑ **Define Your Willingness:**

Understand what you can offer and how much time you can commit.

☑ **Identify Ideal Mentee:**

Determine the qualities you're looking for in a mentee.

☑ Set Clear Boundaries:
Discuss the scope of your mentorship, availability, and methods of communication.

☑ Establish Goals:
Understand your mentee's objectives and how you can assist in achieving them.

☑ Prepare for Meetings:
Consider what advice or resources you can provide to address your mentee's current challenges.

☑ Listen Actively:
Provide a safe space for your mentee to share their thoughts, fears, and aspirations.

☑ Provide Constructive Feedback:
Offer insights and advice that encourage growth and learning.

☑ Monitor Progress:
Keep track of your mentee's development and adjust your guidance as needed.

☑ Encourage Independence:
Empower your mentee to make decisions and learn from their experiences.

☑ Reflect on the Relationship:
Regularly consider how the mentorship is going and what might be improved.

Sample Post-Mentorship Session Checklist

☑ Review the Discussion:
Briefly summarize the key points discussed during the session.

Note any significant advice, insights, or personal revelations.

☑ Evaluate Achievements:
Assess progress made towards the goals set at the beginning of the mentorship or the session.

Acknowledge any accomplishments or improvements, no matter how small.

☑ Reflect on Challenges:
Identify any areas of difficulty or topics that were particularly challenging.

Consider why these were challenging and what can be learned from them.

☑ Plan Action Steps:
List the actions you've agreed to take before the next session.
Be specific about what you will do and by when.

☑ Schedule Next Session:
Agree on a date and time for the next meeting.

Decide on any topics or preparation needed for the next session.

☑ Seek Feedback:

For mentees: Provide feedback to your mentor on what was helpful or what you'd like to see differently.

For mentors: Ask your mentee how they felt about the session and how you can better support them.

☑ Personal Reflection:

Spend a few minutes reflecting on how you felt during the session.

Note any personal growth, changes in perspective, or increased understanding.

☑ Update Learning Log/Journal:

Update your personal learning log or journal with new insights and progress notes.

Include reflections, feelings, and any questions that arose during the session.

☑ Resource Gathering:

If any resources, such as articles, books, or tools, were suggested during the session, list them for follow-up.

Plan when and how you will explore these resources.

☑ Self-Care Check:
Acknowledge the emotional and intellectual energy spent during the session.

Plan some form of self-care to recharge and reflect, such as a walk, meditation, or a hobby.

CHAPTER 12:
SELF-REFLECTION

Having led seminars nationwide, I'm always inclined to take participants through a self-analysis. These steps enable you to see yourself in ten minutes and determine if there is a need for change.

Step 1:

List your top five priorities in order of relevance.

Here's an example:

1. God
2. Family
3. Church
4. Community Service
5. Work

List your top five here:

_____

_____

_____

_____

_____

_____

_____

Step 2:

Draw a clock 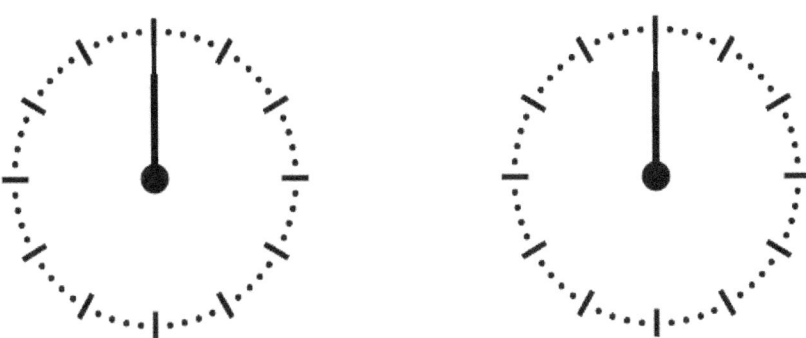 that represents twenty-four hours with times listed.

Identify when you are sleeping, awake, working, preparing for work, doing community service, in traffic, etc. In a twenty-four-hour period list how much time you spend in each area.

Out of twenty-four hours in a day how much time in a day, week, or month do you spend on your top priorities?

_____

_____

_____

_____

After looking at your response, remember you have a choice. How do you spend your time and what does it say about you?

_____

_____

_____

_____

Self-analysis: What is your definition of success in your personal and professional life?

_____

_____

_____

_____

If you are in an organization to serve the community, how much time do you spend serving those in need?

_____

_____

_____

_____

Does your purpose in life allow you to live a life of purpose?

_____

_____

_____

_____

How much time do you spend in email wars, meetings, and deciding what position you will hold in the upcoming election versus fulfilling the actual mission of the organization?

_____

_____

_____

_____

If you are in an organization for your children, do your children enjoy the activities, or have you made the time about you?

_____

_____

_____

_____

Your family wants you, your time, and your focus. Do you give it to them?

_____

_____

_____

_____

The majority of women I have interviewed who complete the wheel spend their time in reverse order. In essence, you say your priorities are God, Family, Church, Community Service, and Work; however, where you invest your time says your priorities are Work, Community Service, Church, Family, and God. You must create balance.

Creating Balance and Understanding Support Systems

How can those we care for find their purpose and balance when we don't have ours?

_____

_____

_____

_____

Are you "Ms. I must have it now?"

Patience is a necessity. Everything that's meant for the next person may not be meant for you. When you find your purpose, you find your direction. Be prepared, but be patient.

Are you "Ms. Calm your mind?"

Rest, meditation, and focus should be part of your normal routine. In reading this book, how many times did you answer the phone, look at a computer, or respond to the needs of someone else? Often our lives are so full of distractions that we can't enjoy the moment that we are in.

To create balance, you must be held accountable for your actions.

Find an accountability partner. The only requirement for an accountability partner is that they not tell you what you want to hear, but what you need to hear. But how is this different from having a mentor?

Understanding the Difference: Accountability Partner vs. Mentor

An accountability partner and a mentor serve different roles in your growth and development:

Accountability Partner: Typically a peer, this person helps keep you focused on specific, short-term goals through regular check-ins. This relationship is often reciprocal, with both parties holding each other accountable.

Mentor: Usually someone with more experience, a mentor provides long-term guidance and support, helping you navigate broader personal and professional growth. This relationship is more one-way, with the mentor offering their wisdom and experience. *Go back to Chapter 11 to review this concept.*

Recognizing whether you need an accountability partner, a mentor, or both can help you seek the right kind of support at different times in your life. Both can play a crucial role in your journey toward balance and fulfillment.

Accountability Partner Checklist:

- Identify Your Ideal Partner:
  Look for someone who is honest, constructive, and genuinely interested in your growth.

- Set Clear Expectations:
  Discuss the frequency of meetings, the method of communication, and the specific areas where you need accountability.

- Establish Goals and Milestones:
  Clearly outline what you aim to achieve with their support and set realistic deadlines.

- Communication Plan:
  Decide how you will share updates and feedback, whether through regular meetings, calls, or messages.

- Feedback and Adjustment:
  Be open to receiving honest feedback and willing to adjust your strategies as needed.

- Celebrate Successes:
  Acknowledge every achievement, no matter how small, and share these moments with your partner.

- Addressing Challenges:
  Discuss any obstacles you're facing and seek advice on how to overcome them.

- Regular Review:
  Periodically assess the effectiveness of the partnership and make adjustments where necessary.

The Problem

We have allowed ourselves to come to a place of complacency with the health disparities that are plaguing our communities. If we aren't in our best physical and emotional health, we are compromising the gifts that each of us gives and brings. We are overworked and overwhelmed to the point that nothing is occurring.

Take time each day to make sure that you have committed to ensuring that your own internal and physical house is in order before trying to fix someone else's home. Your community starts in your own home.

To pretend that we live in perfection is a misconception and an ongoing problem that has devastating consequences. Rarely do people get everything right the first time. The opportunity to learn, unlearn, and relearn can be a powerful experience. Celebrate your success along the way. Take time to determine what works well for you and to release what hinders you. Below are some additional tools to help you.

Additional Tools:

- **Set Aside Time:**
  Dedicate a quiet, uninterrupted time each day. Consider this an investment in your personal growth and balance.

- **Reflective Mindset:**
  Be honest with yourself about where you currently stand and where you want to be.

- **Self-Reflection:**
  Assess your current state of being. Contemplate your definition of success and how it aligns with your daily life.

- **Time Management:**
  Evaluate and improve how you allocate your time. Think about ways you can make more efficient use of your time to focus on what truly matters.

- **Goal Setting:**
  Setting clear, achievable goals is crucial to personal and professional development. Ensure your goals are well-

defined and aligned with your purpose. Regularly review and adjust them as needed.

- **Well-being and Self-Care:**
  Your physical and mental health are the foundation of a balanced life. Be intentional about taking care of yourself. Make adjustments to your routine as necessary to improve your well-being.

- **Action Steps:**
  Write down specific actions you plan to take based on your reflections. These can be small steps or larger plans, but they should be concrete and achievable.

- **Regular Review:**
  Track your progress toward your goals and make ongoing adjustments. Your needs and circumstances may change over time, and your approach should evolve accordingly.

- **Seek Support:**
  If you find areas where you're struggling or need extra help, consider seeking support from a trusted friend, family member, professional, mentor or accountability partner. Sometimes, an outside perspective can provide valuable insights and encouragement.

- **Celebrate Progress:**
  Acknowledge and celebrate any progress you make, no matter how small. All progress is important. Recognizing

your achievements will motivate you to continue working towards your goals and maintaining balance.

These are tools to guide you on your path to a balanced and fulfilled life. They are not meant to be one-time exercises but rather part of an ongoing practice of self-reflection and improvement. Adjust them as needed to fit your unique journey. Let's go deeper.

Self-Reflection:
- Ask yourself:
  Have I clearly defined what success means to me?

  Do my daily activities align with my top five priorities?

  Am I investing time in relationships and activities that reflect my true values?

  Have I identified areas in my life where imbalance occurs most frequently?

  What steps can I take to reduce stress and increase fulfillment in my daily life?

Time Management:
- Time management is a key to success.
- Ask yourself:

  Have I identified my most productive times of the day?
  Do I have a clear schedule that allocates time for work, rest, and personal growth?

Have I set realistic goals for what I can achieve in a day/ week/month?

Am I regularly reviewing and adjusting my schedule to prevent overcommitment?

Do I delegate tasks when possible to maintain a balanced workload?

Goal Setting:

- Have you set goals? Are the goals identified:

  - Realistic: Are my goals realistic and within reach given my current resources and constraints?

  - Understandable: Have I clearly articulated my goals so they are easy to understand and communicate to others if needed?

  - Measurable: Can I track and measure my progress towards these goals?
    - What benchmarks can I set to know I'm moving in the right direction?

  - Behavioral: Do these goals encourage positive behavior changes or actions that I can consistently perform and maintain over time?

  - Attainable: Are these goals challenging yet achievable?

◆ Do they stretch my abilities without being so lofty that they become discouraging?

❯ Have I written down my goals and reviewed them regularly?

❯ Do I have a plan for overcoming potential obstacles to achieving my goals?

❯ Am I tracking my progress and celebrating small victories along the way?

- Do I regularly reflect on and adjust my goals as needed?

Well-being and Self-Care:
- Your health matters! Ask yourself:
  ❯ Am I getting enough sleep and rest?

  ❯ Do I have a regular exercise routine that I enjoy?

  ❯ Am I eating a balanced and nutritious diet?

- Do I have stress-reduction techniques that work for me (e.g., meditation, journaling)?

- Do I make time for hobbies and activities that bring me joy?

Final Thoughts

Understanding your purpose and creating balance isn't a one-time act but a continuous process. Revisit these steps and questions regularly. Reflect on your progress and be open to adjusting your path as you evolve. Your path to a balanced and fulfilling life is uniquely yours. Embrace it with patience, understanding, and a relentless commitment to living a life that truly reflects who you are and what you value most.

CHAPTER 13

SHARED STORIES

The FIT Concept: A Universal Tool for Balance. The FIT concept is a tool I created to encourage people to take an opportunity to focus on Family, Internal self, and Time. It allows people to adapt it for each individual's unique circumstances and interpersonal goals. Whether you're single, married, a parent, a student, or at any other stage of life, FIT is about balancing the critical aspects of your life in a way that resonates with your situation and values.

Family (F): Family refers to the connections that support and enrich your life, whether they are biological relatives, close friends, or community members. It's about nurturing the relationships that bring you joy and stability.

- Schedule regular device-free family dinners. Use this time to connect and communicate openly with your loved ones.
- Engage in meaningful activities with those you consider family, like friends or community groups. Organize regular outings or participate in group activities that foster connection.

Internal (I): Taking time for internal reflection and self-care is crucial for everyone. It's about understanding and attending to your mental, emotional, and physical needs.

- Incorporate activities like meditation, journaling, or physical exercise into your routine. Find what centers you and make it a non-negotiable part of your day.

Time (T): Managing your time effectively is universal. It's about setting boundaries and priorities to create a balanced and fulfilling life.

- Assess your commitments and be honest about what brings value to your life. Be selective about your commitments, choosing only what aligns with your values and brings you joy.

Success Stories

1. *Before I understood the FIT concept, my life was a flurry of missed moments and unfulfilled commitments. After ensuring regular family dinners and dedicating time for self-care, my relationships strengthened, and I felt more centered. FIT became my way of reclaiming my life.*

2. *I've always seen myself as independent, but the FIT concept made me realize that independence doesn't mean isolation. I started viewing my close friends and community as my Family. These changes didn't just improve my life; they enhanced the quality of every minute I lived.*

Answer the following questions to explore your FIT level. How do you spend your time?

_____

_____

_____

_____

_____

- With whom do you spend your time?

_____

_____

_____

_____

- Are you a member of the drive-thru ministry? i.e., Are you eating meals on the go in your car instead of having sit-down dinners with your family or even yourself alone at home?

_____

_____

_____

_____

- Do you make time for family dinners to talk with your children about their day at school? How about dinner with your friends, family, or simply a quiet moment of reflection by yourself?

_____

_____

_____

_____

_____

- Are you on Internet sites or using mobile devices when your family needs your uninterrupted attention?

_____

_____

_____

_____

_____

- Do you communicate with your children or family through the intercom of the house or on electronic devices when you are in the room next to them?

_____

_____

_____

_____

_____

Transitioning from the foundational upbringing many women receive from their mothers or maternal figures, where they are often taught the roles of a wife, mother, caregiver, or even household responsibilities like cooking, there is a transition into the development of habits and routines that stem from these early lessons. This ingrained upbringing frequently leads to women becoming adept at juggling multiple responsibilities, including life, family, and work. The emphasis on prioritizing the needs of others often comes at the expense of their own well-being becomes a habit.

Roles, Habits, and Routines

Roles:
- Wife: Partner and supporter.
- Mother: Caregiver and nurturer.
- Daughter/Sister: Support system and confidant.
- Friend: Companion and ally.

_____

_____

_____

_____

Habits:
- Prioritizing others' needs over one's own.
- Multi-tasking daily responsibilities.
- Seeking perfection and order in various life aspects.

_____

_____

_____

_____

_____

Routines:

- Daily rituals for managing household, career, and relationships.

- Scheduled self-care (often neglected).

- Balancing social life with personal and family time.

_____

_____

_____

_____

Historically, some women made home the priority. Now there are women who spend their days with happy hours, meetings, and social engagements. The dangerous part about computers and social media sites is that people can create the image of being a happy family member rather than living the real image of what they portray. In today's society, you cannot believe everything that you see online or on television.

Jealousy and envy can develop when you spend too much time focusing on what your image looks like in comparison to others rather than living the life you have been blessed to live. Do not allow jealousy to rob you of enjoying all of the blessings that you already have.

However, one must ask the question, where are your loved ones and family while you are at the meetings?

_____

_____

_____

_____

Where is your family when you are creating optics of happiness?

_____

_____

_____

_____

Is the meeting worth the sacrifice?

_____

_____

_____

_____

What are you doing in your everyday life to satisfy you?

_____

_____

_____

_____

Why does it take returning for you to decide, "I'm going to take a bath and satisfy my mind for an hour," when you could have been satisfying your mind all day?

_____

_____

_____

_____

Instead of gathering friends to join you at the gym, do you go for a walk in the park (for free) with your children, spouse, or significant other?

_____

_____

_____

_____

Do you spend time with yourself?

_____

_____

_____

_____

Reflect on a time when you felt imbalanced. What were the contributing factors, and how could applying the FIT principle have helped?

_____

_____

_____

_____

Consider your answers to the questions above and identify one change you could make to improve your balance.

The Impact

Time for self must become the priority before time for others. There is an ongoing breakdown that has contributed to a worldwide epidemic among women. An honest assessment is the starting point. It is impossible to break through imbalance unless we are honest that a breakdown has occurred and we take time to observe the breakdown. In life, we don't see things the way they are. It is through our own lens and experiences that we see and shape things the way they are.

You must have a firm belief in yourself before you have belief in others. Without this, your existence is unproductive and through the lens of others who will always view you the way they are, not the way you are. It is important to have a strong sense of self and that sense of self cannot be contingent upon what other people think about you.

Over the years I have found women operating at minimal levels, low capacity, and regardless of how good the external appearance looked, many were on the verge of a mental, physical, emotional, and psychological meltdown. Often, only by slowing down can the true speed of one's momentum be realized; especially if it was previously unrecognized. A high need for external gratification and placing oneself in stressful positions often contribute to neglecting excellent self-care.

Nutrition has been compromised. We exist in a society that overeating, have forgotten portion control, and the need for immediate gratification has led many of us to meals on the go. Taking time to meditate, exercise, and get regular health exams has become an afterthought. Slow down and listen to your body, what does it need? Water, movement, rest? Take care of yourself, do not let your health be an afterthought. In order to do this, please allow me to introduce you to the FIT Concept: A Universal Tool for Balance.

Final Thoughts

Remember that the FIT concept is not about fitting your life into predefined categories but about shaping these categories to fit your life. Reflect on how Family, Internal self, and Time manifest for you, and tailor your approach to nurture a balanced, fulfilling existence. Your journey is yours, and so is your version of FIT. Embrace it with patience, understanding, and a relentless commitment to living a life that truly reflects who you are and what you value most.

Whether you live a life of balance or imbalance, the choice is yours.

CHAPTER 14

SACRIFICE, ENDURANCE, GOALS

"I was someone who said yes to everything. Driven by a deep-seated need to be liked and feared loneliness so intensely that I surrounded myself with people constantly. However, these relationships weren't always genuine. I stretched myself thin, trying to be everything to everyone, which led to panic attacks, grief, and a profound loss of self. I had morphed into everything others wanted me to be and, in the process, lost sight of who I truly was. I was imbalanced inside but to the world I was balanced and successful. It was time for a change. It was only when I found the word no that things began to change and get better."

There are many things that lead to imbalance, so discussing sacrifice, endurance, and goals is essential. Exploring how the interplay of sacrifice, endurance, and goal-setting can either exacerbate or mitigate feelings of imbalance in the lives of women, offering pathways to deeper fulfillment. By understanding and applying the principles discussed, you can navigate the complexities of life with greater clarity, purpose, and balance.

Sacrifice

When you say yes to something that is not related to your goals, it will require a sacrifice and only you can determine if it is a sacrifice worth making. You can sacrifice yourself, have great endurance, and be successful, however if this does not align with your personal goals you can eventually find yourself in a place of imbalance. Often, the sacrifices made in pursuit of success or approval from others can lead us away from what truly matters in our lives. The pressure to meet external expectations can overshadow our own values and priorities, resulting in a profound sense of imbalance.

An example of this is seen in the life of an obstetrician who faced a choice between her professional duties and her family. She felt she was always prioritizing her patients, often missing out on family moments so that she could be present to assist in delivering her patients' babies. When her daughter's ballet recital came up, and her daughter really wanted her not to miss it as she usually did due to work, she faced a tough decision. This was new for her and initially a tough choice. Choosing her daughter this time, she stepped back from work, letting her team cover. This rare choice to put family first, despite her deep sense of duty to her patients, was a significant step in finding a balance between her professional obligations and personal life. For the first time, she removed the eternal pressure of being there for everyone else and sacrificing her family. It was the first step in many, and as her family life benefitted from this new behavior, she realized this was a habit that she wanted to keep.

Beyond personal choices, our behaviors around sacrifice are often shaped by societal expectations and learned behaviors. There are learned behaviors for example where we have been trained to make sacrifices by forfeiting ourselves and family time for false images and perceptions. Do you need a title to be a good mother, daughter, sister, aunt, or friend? Do you need a title to be a good person? Of course not. An important lesson to learn is how to stop adding meetings, titles, events, and organizations to your agenda for fear of using the word "no" especially when adding this causes you imbalance. You don't have to be everything to everyone.

Remember, the word "no" can be a complete sentence. In many instances the word "no" is just as powerful as "yes." In the search for balance and fulfillment, learning the value and use of the word "no" can be transformative.

To have balance you must learn to embrace the word "no." In fact, you must learn to love the word "no." Then you must learn to use the word "no." While understanding the power of "no" is crucial, equally important is how we endure the challenges life throws our way, shaping our journey towards balance.

Endurance

Endurance can be viewed as the ability to sustain a prolonged activity or effort. We admire those who push through adversity, often without considering the toll it takes on their health and happiness. However, this traditional view of endurance can lead to a tolerance for situations that are not just challenging but extremely harmful.

Building endurance to tolerate adverse situations doesn't necessarily mean we're focusing our efforts on what truly matters or investing time in things we should be doing

The best way to demonstrate and promote healthy endurance and translate a message of health and wellness to your sons, daughters, spouses, family, and community is to involve them in becoming their own health advocates through health and wellness initiatives. People do what they see us do, not what we tell them to do.

True endurance isn't about gritting our teeth through toxic situations but about persisting in practices that align with our well-being, such as regular self-care and setting realistic expectations. This redefined approach encourages us not just to survive but to thrive, ensuring that the challenges we face don't compromise our health and happiness.

It is imperative that you make time for health related activities including screenings, eye exams, dental exams, physicals, exercise, etc. If you don't take care of your body, where do you plan to live? Many people look good on the outside but can be unhealthy on the inside. Imbalance can occur when we build up endurance to do things that we think we should be doing that do not align with our purpose or distract us from taking care of our health. With a sustainable approach to endurance in our toolkit, setting and pursuing clear goals becomes the next step in guiding us toward responding to daily commitments and priorities.

Goals

It's time to do better. The only way to do better is to have direction and purpose. If you do not know the direction to where you are going, chances are you may never get there. Goals are the purpose that provide directions that can help navigate you on your path in life. Without goals there is a risk of aimless wandering, which eventually leads to a place of imbalance.

Goals are the ingredients for life's recipe, even if that means a choice to change. Effective goals are well-written goals that are detailed and measurable. If you have an accountability partner let them know your goal(s) and make sure s/he/they understand the importance of holding you accountable.

However, even with clear goals, we may encounter obstacles such as losing motivation or facing unexpected setbacks. The journey toward achieving our goals is not always smooth. It's important to recognize these challenges and develop strategies to overcome them. Breaking goals into smaller, achievable tasks can help maintain momentum and make the process less intimidating. Additionally, building a support system of friends, family, or mentors who understand and support your goals can provide the encouragement and accountability needed during challenging times.

Knowing your goals can impact how you start your day. Each morning, start your day by determining one thing that you can do today, to make you better for your tomorrow. The most effective tool for personal growth begins with honest and quiet reflection on one's own life.

Once you identify your recipe for change, by setting goals, you must begin implementation. Keep in mind that words have power and can support or derail your progress. Make a **list** of words and statements that empower you as a reminder of things you value, what you're trying to achieve, and why it's important to stay positive and have balance. Consider the following examples of strategies that can promote balance:

- Speak life and maintain positive thoughts.

- Don't focus on external validation to the point where you don't focus on you.

- Every decision that you make in life does not require the affirmation or approval of other people.

- Be happy for yourself.

- It's wonderful to celebrate your success and be proud of your own accomplishments.

- Your words matter. Manifest a positive future for yourself. Just because three generations of your family before you had heart disease, doesn't mean that you will or have to have a similar diagnosis.

- Make a conscious choice to expect to live a long, healthy, and prosperous life.

- Keep positive people close to you.

- Put resources in place to remain FIT and balanced.

- Eat healthy, go for walks, exercise, and stay active.

- Commit to taking care of yourself as a priority.

  You are worth it.

- Make time for you and be the change that you want to see.

Set Boundaries

Reflect on how to manage the opportunities and responsibilities that you are presented with; understanding that every opportunity is not always meant to be pursued. If patience is a virtue, then you must accept the fact that everything that comes to you is not always for you. The opportunities that come to you and pass you are meant to go somewhere else. Have peace in knowing this. Sometimes you have to stay in your lane and be comfortable with what you have right in front of you. Imbalance can occur when you think that every available opportunity is for you. Every title and position is not for you. Therefore it is important to understand the beauty of blessing others by cheering them on for the great things that are being accomplished in their lives.

Don't be afraid to train others for leadership and be an advocate for their success even if it is in an opportunity that passed you by or that you passed on. Just because a moment of overflow is not for you doesn't mean you can't steer that opportunity towards another well qualified person. This may not apply to you yet it is disconcerting to me that it is easier for someone to help a stranger rather than help a colleague in need. This is also a sign of imbalance.

You have to be in a certain mindset to have balance. Why is it uncomfortable for many women to be still? You don't always have to chase the wind as it never stops blowing. The right things will come to you when you hold still. In society, success is often correlated to how busy day planners are, the number of organizations you are a member of, and how many titles or degrees that can be added to your signature block.

"At one point in my life, I was a member of the most prestigious women's leadership and service organizations and held local, national, and regional titles. My day planner was full—almost every weekend with a flight/conference/meeting – as many accolades donned my walls. I thought these things were successful steps in life based on observations of the women who I thought were successful, but I never achieved the end goal of peace and

being able to enjoy my family. I had a family meeting in my house and apologized for being too busy for those I loved. I haven't looked back nor allowed anything to be my priority except for those that truly are the priority."

Have you had a family meeting recently? Even if you are not married, have a family meeting with those closest to you. Do you know the impact that each family member has on the other? Consider parents: Have you filled your children's day with school and activities to the point where they can't enjoy life and have increased stress? Are those in your family unit too busy to enjoy life or time with you?

_____

_____

_____

_____

_____

_____

_____

_____

_____

Women who view and measure success as being busy may create children, families, mentees, and others in society who do the same. Is there an unhealthy and unproductive imbalanced cycle being created in your home or life? Consider today the day that you make a difference by making a change for the better.

An attendee at a workshop I held defined success as "the ability to accomplish goals that you set for yourself without compromising your integrity and happiness."

Only you know how you will measure success, what areas of your life need to be enhanced, and how to develop a better balance for yourself, your family, and those whose lives you impact. Take time to focus on how you feel more than what you see. If your daily schedule is overflowing, it may appear successful, but if the thought of completing every task in a day overwhelms you, consider what can be postponed to create a balanced and enjoyable day that suits your needs.

Redefining Relationships

Do you remember Sally who you read about earlier? Things turned out well for her. In her world, she shares that success starts with God and starts at home. She wasn't a success until her end goal correlated with her priority list. None of the women who she thought were successful taught her that. In fact, once she made the great epiphany and transition, the tables turned and she became a mentor to the women who she initially held in such high esteem and strived to be like. Mutual mentorship can be positive when expectations are clearly defined and also when both people realize that each person may have contributions that can enhance the relationship.

Contributions Extend Beyond Monetary Moments

She values their relationships and respects them even more for their openness with her and for their ability to follow her lead now puts family first and allows mutual mentorship. To some success is that they may have exceeded her financially in salaries at some points in her career, but currently, she has found the success points as the places where she exceeds them in having balance. This is priceless.

Overextending as Related to External Commitments

Are you a successful failure? Your mindset and priority list will determine what success is for you. Women are at risk of losing sight of their personal priorities because they are talented and successful in organizations and work. This isn't to say that one should abstain from leadership positions in organizations. However, when such leadership positions start to eclipse one's home life and consume the majority of one's time, it can lead to imbalance, strained family relationships, and often negatively impact marriages and other personal connections. If you are unhappy, resign so that you can replenish the reservoir of happiness in your life.

Imbalance can cause us to be successful failures.

"Like many, I have learned from experience. Currently, I'm only in a few organizations whose missions I strongly believe in. I've developed a 90-minute limit on meetings from the scheduled start time; then I go home to my family. If the meeting starts late, that does not mean that I am obligated to stay late.

I encourage you to determine your limits, set goals, and stick to them. The meeting isn't your priority; your family is. Don't be afraid to keep your balance and go home."

We must determine if we are in organizations because we

think they will help us in our careers or because we truly believe in the mission statement of the organization. Sometimes being in an organization requires sacrifice of one's family life, personal balance, and mental health; only you can determine if it's worth the sacrifice for you. When meetings extend into dinner time with family, are you disciplined enough to have a limit and cut-off time to know when it's time for you to go home?

What methods of balance will you utilize in your life that will allow you to make sustainable changes for your balance in the future? Every day that we have is a gift that cannot be replaced. What will you do to show your appreciation for the gift that you have been given? Who will you show this appreciation to and why? Will you show it to your family and to the source that has granted you the breath of life?

Reflect on life

What advice would you give your twenty-year-old self? If you are in your twenties, what advice would you have given yourself five to ten years ago? Often we look back and appreciate where we were and what we had after it is gone. In this current moment what can you learn from past experiences that can help you make wise decisions for any challenges you are facing?

_____

_____

_____

_____

_____

_____

Actionable Tip: Reflect on Your 'Yes' and Your 'No'

This week, practice saying "no" to something that doesn't align with your priorities or well-being. Notice how it feels to assert your boundaries and reflect on the extra time or peace of mind you gain as a result. Think about a recent time you said "yes" when you really wanted to say "no". What were the consequences, and how did it make you feel about yourself and your time?

Embracing NO is the first step in truly understanding and asserting your value. It's not just a word; it's a declaration of your priorities and your right to choose. Choose YOU!

Embrace An Affirmation That Protects Your Peace

Verbalize the following statement daily until it manifests into an outcome that restores your balance and peace:

I am entitled to my time and energy.

I will say "no" when it protects my peace and respects my well-being.

This affirmation is an important reminder to reemphasize that saying "no" can be empowering and its utilization is essential for maintaining balance. While it is true that sacrifice is a frequently necessary component of many endeavors, this shouldn't come at the cost of your health and happiness. Remember that endurance is about more than pushing through; it's also about knowing when to rest. Goals should align with your values and contribute to your well-being and incorporate rest when needed.

Overflow happens, and is a recurring theme in life but you must control how it affects you and what you allow into your life. Understanding your true self is the key to genuine success and fulfillment.

Final Thoughts

Sacrifice, endurance, and goal-setting intertwine to guide us through what many describe as the maze of our existence. Embracing sacrifice with awareness, considering when to use the strength of endurance, and choosing your course having clear goals, are not merely about surviving, but thriving, while making the shift from feeling overwhelmed to achieving an equilibrium. This is what shifts from imbalance to balance, and it is liberating.

With the concepts of sacrifice, endurance, and goals, a comprehensive picture of the balancing act evolves. Vital tools such as saying "no" can be just as significant as saying "Yes." Once you understand this concept, you are equipped to impact your path to fulfillment and balance. Reflect on your own life and the times you've said yes to others at the expense of your well-being. It's time to assert your value and prioritize your needs.

My hope is that you will embrace the journey with an open heart and mind, and let each step, each reflection, and each moment of honesty bring you closer to the life you're meant to live; a life filled with purpose, joy, and balance. Your life is a precious gift, and how you choose to spend it is entirely up to you. Make decisions that bring you good health and peace. In embracing these principles, you have the power and opportunity to redefine what it means to lead a balanced and fulfilled life. Balance must be a priority.

CHAPTER 15:
BUSY TRAP

At the conclusion of a presentation for a national seminar, one of the participants approached me with tears in her eyes and said, "I want to step back from all of these leadership positions, but I don't know how. What will they think of me?" When we redirected the discussion to the priority list that she had just completed in the seminar and asked what her priorities were she said, "God, husband, children, church, work, and organizations."

She further explained, "Everything you said makes sense. This seminar has changed my life. I want to change, but I'm afraid. I feel trapped. I'm a national officer; what am I supposed to do? My marriage is now in turmoil, my children say I don't spend time with them, and the only success I have is in this organization and at work."

Do you get caught in the "busy trap" looking to please others? We all have a trigger. What is your trigger that causes you to be in situations that overwhelm you, situations where you said you would say no but you find yourself doing that which you do not want to do?

_____

_____

_____

_____

_____

_____

Are you in a state where everything feels as if it is moving in fast forward? Are you racing through the day, missing all of the beautiful moments in life? Do you rush from meeting to meeting, from event to event, from phone call to phone call, or from social media site to social media site? How are you spending your time?

_____

_____

_____

_____

_____

Knowing what you know now, look back over the pattern of your life when you were most imbalanced. What advice would you give to your busy self, the overwhelmed self, or the unhappy self? Don't be critical, be honest, and elaborate, but end with supportive thoughts to know that you are SAFE. Write them down.

_____

_____

_____

_____

_____

_____

_____

_____

_____

_____

_____

_____

_____

_____

_____

To date, I have not seen a priority list where an organization or work is listed above religion and family, yet organizations and work steal time from things we list as priorities.

When you are at a meeting and struggling to leave, pull out a mirror, look in it and determine who you love more. Do you love the person in the mirror? Is she, the person looking back at you in the mirror, happy at this moment in time? If not, pack your items and leave.

The rationale for this mindset is simple: you must get to the source of the problem. To be everything to others and nothing to self is like an ulcer untreated; it's going to get worse unless you treat it. You could assume that if more women knew how to have peace choosing our priorities, and set a parameter of when to go home, meetings would run more effectively and end sooner. The only person left in the room would be the person who has nothing else to do; and that person would not be you. People cannot abuse your time if you do not allow them to.

"I've learned that I can lose money and earn it again, but when I give you my time, that's a gift that can never be earned again. Everyone is not worthy of the gift of your time; be careful who you give it to."

Power of Journaling

Journaling is an effective tool to identify moments of imbalance. When you journal, include the time along with the other information; it's an effective way to see where you are at a moment in time. When you look back you can see if you have made progress, regression, or are at a place of stagnation. This is an important part of maintaining balance.

"Looking back through a journal entry I wrote at 3:55 a.m. on a night energized with insomnia I wrote the following: For one day she doesn't want to be needed by anyone. Everyone says, "It will be okay, you're fine," yet she fights to be the glue that holds everything together.

For one day she doesn't want to be needed by anyone. She will give the world to put a smile on the faces of those that she loves but often fails to know how to put a smile on her own face.

For one day she doesn't want to be needed by anyone. Just a day of rest, relaxation, and solitude. To explore the moon and the stars. To see the sun glimmer in all of its essence.

To smell the sweet scent in the air after the rain. To look in the Solarium and gaze at all of the possibilities in the sky. For one day she doesn't want to be needed by anyone.

Unfortunately, that day seems a long way from coming."

At the moment above, I was tired. I remember thinking, I'm so tired, I want to be everything to everyone, but I need to do some things for me. This exhausting moment taught me the importance of a detox. I call this an imbalance detox.

What is an imbalance detox and why should you detox?

Sometimes you have to detox from what you thought was good for your mind and body to find out that it really was not good for you at all. What areas of your life need to be detoxed today? Let's be very clear: I am speaking of more than food. Sometimes a mental, physical, emotional, and psychological detox is needed. Remove all of the harmful substances and people from your life. No one is off limits. Again, I ask you what areas of your life need to be detoxed today? Write them here.

_____

_____

_____

_____

_____

_____

_____

_____

_____

_____

_____

_____

As you begin to detox, consider using affirmations to assist you in staying focused on what the detox is removing and why it matters. The following sample affirmations can be beneficial. As a reminder, recite each one out loud daily.

- I prioritize what truly matters in my life: family, faith, and personal well-being.
- I am in control of my time, and I choose to invest it wisely.
- I am confident in setting boundaries and saying no when necessary.
- I am deserving of balance and harmony in my life.
- I value my mental and emotional well-being above all else.

Mental Eviction Notice

After the detox it's time for a term I coined called a *Mental Eviction Notice*. A mental eviction notice is defined as making a firm decision to have peace with things, people, and organizations that you must let go of. It is important to evict negative energy and people from your life. Knowing when it is time to release people, organizations, and negative situations from your life can initially be challenging. You may feel a sense of loyalty. You may even feel that if you do not remain in your current role, no one else will step up and take your place. Guilt and being consumed by what others think can cause you to be imbalanced.

How you feel physically and emotionally after interacting with people is also a sign for knowing when you are in a state of balance or imbalance. For example, if it consistently takes you two hours to calm down from conversations with specific individuals or from attending a meeting, these may be areas that you must evict from your life. We are emblematic of the health concerns of the future. How are you living your life? If your community lived your life the way that you live your life, what would your community look like? In other words, would you live in a community of fear or peace, order or confusion, growth or stagnation, health or ailment?

_____

_____

_____

_____

_____

_____

_____

_____

_____

_____

_____

_____

_____

_____

_____

_____

Inner Harmony

Women who feel chaos create communities of chaos. Women who feel conflicted embrace conflict. This is because hurt people hurt other people. Do you love the person in the mirror? Achieving inner harmony is an intentional act. You must have mental clarity. Your peace of mind is your most precious gift. When you develop the ability to have mental peace of mind among any chaotic storm that approaches you, you are in a powerful place. No one can steal your joy. It is only you who can allow another person to take your joy away. Poor mental health creates physical stress. We can only attract what we are good at by being in harmony.

Often Achieving your being and purpose will require you to dial back on the noise of distractions and focus on you. When this time comes, and it will, remember your detox. Below is a checklist to give you ideas to give you some steps on the road to an effective detox.

Detox Checklist

☑ Identify areas of your life that may need detoxification.

☑ Consider physical detox, including dietary changes if necessary.

☑ Reflect on mental, emotional, and psychological aspects that require detox.

☑ List harmful substances or negative influences that should be removed.

☑ Make a firm decision to prioritize peace and well-being.

☑ Evaluate the impact of your lifestyle on your community.

☑ Recognize the importance of mental clarity and peace of mind.

☑ Embrace the power of maintaining your peace and joy.

☑ Understand the connection between mental health and physical well-being.

Final Thoughts

Setting priorities, learning to say no, and maintaining mental clarity are keys to a fulfilling life. Detox not just your body but your mind and emotions too. Evict negativity and embrace positivity. Your journey to balance and self-care is a gift to yourself that you deserve.

CHAPTER 16:
AUTHENTIC CONVERSATION

Experiencing pain, joy, love, happiness, and sorrow shapes our stories, leaving us with experiences ready to be shared with others. I have always hoped that I would be strong enough to embrace the power of vulnerability, to allow myself to be the light at the end of the tunnel to help others know that light exists within them. My hope is that you join me.

We are each special in our own way and we must allow our light to shine bright, so that we can offer guidance for others to discover their glow without delay. The more balanced and empowered we are, the more we can do this for others. Our experiences are like ties that bind us—let's support one another, symbolically locking in arms in unity with an unspoken commitment to sparing each other unnecessary pain. The next generation must be left with a footprint in the sand heading in the right direction, and an example to show them the possibilities that exist, as well as the impossibilities that exist when they don't care for themselves.

True success originates from how we feel the internal positive questions originating from within, not from external accolades or achievements. The construct of success must **not** encompass competitiveness, divisiveness, and arrogance against another person. These negative emotions and characteristics evolve when there is fear and insecurity. This is why balance is important. Balanced individuals create harmonious communities, radiating and attracting positivity. Balanced people attract other positive people and contribute to making the world we live in a better place.

We all have a place and seat at the table that is unique to us, that was created for us, and whose impactful and rewarding contributions can only be made by us. We do not have to sit at every table harboring envy, jealousy, and hatred in our hearts. When we prioritize and work together with others in harmony and peace, the universe honors us and great things happen.

In writing this book, it became apparent to me that for many women, there is no endpoint. We constantly add ingredients to ourselves. Once we finish one recipe–in essence, a life goal–we begin to search for the next recipe to add to our menu called life. There must be a stopping point, a point where you recognize you are good enough. Many women struggle with this. Well, you are good enough, you are powerful, resilient, and deserving of love, peace, happiness, and joy.

Personal Reflection

As I continue to reflect on my own journey, I've encountered moments of self-doubt and uncertainty. It was in those moments that I discovered the strength within me to persevere. I realized that I am good enough, just as you are. Embrace your uniqueness, your power, and your worth.

Encouragement

Today, take a moment for yourself. Acknowledge your strength, resilience, and the love that resides within you. You have the capacity to create positive change.

Call to Action

Take action. Prioritize self-care and set boundaries. The journey to finding balance, or falling into imbalance, works like a muscle that gets stronger over time. Like a muscle, both balance and imbalance will get used to certain behaviors, via your everyday actions and choices that shape you. Using the muscle of your choice (balance or imbalance) you are either building up your strength and enjoying balance or being worn down creating imbalance. The more you use the muscle of balance through repetition, the stronger it gets, the choice is yours.

Always pay attention to habits, because they decide whether you are building up your ability to stay balanced or making it easier to move into imbalance. The trouble comes when daily habits lean more towards imbalance, throwing you off of balance. Intentionally consider areas to create and maintain balance, and make them a priority. Revisit the content in this book often as you continue on your daily journey of genuine fulfillment and maintaining balance.

Each chapter you've explored, each question you've answered, and each moment of introspection and growth you've engaged in demonstrates your willingness to show up in your own life. Keep moving forward, continue working for your balance even though it may not look like a stereotypical norm. Knowing what works for you is not a weakness. In fact it is one of the greatest measures of courage you can demonstrate. Choose YOU! The pursuit of balance leads to a fulfilled life.

Hopefully you are reflecting and thinking in a different way which is what this book is designed to do. Good work!

APPENDIX

Congratulations on taking the next step in your journey with "Imbalance: The Perception of Unfulfillment in the Modern Day Woman." This book is a path for deeper reflection, discussion, and personal growth. Whether you are using this workbook in a book club, within a mastermind group, or in the solitude of personal reflection, if you put in the time and commitment to read, reflect, and renew you shall begin the steps of moving from imbalance towards a more fulfilling and balanced life.

Effective Use For This Book

This book is organized around key themes that resonate with the modern-day woman's goal for fulfillment while battling perceived imbalance. It can be used in many spaces and many formats. Make sure every participant has their own copy to get started.

For Book Clubs: It is structured to facilitate engaging conversations, enabling members to connect the book's themes with their own experiences and societal observations. The thought-provoking questions and activities are designed to enrich your discussions and enhance your collective understanding.

For Mastermind Groups: Mastermind groups focused on personal development and collective empowerment can provide a structured approach to exploring the themes of "Imbalance," encouraging members to share insights, challenges, and breakthroughs. Together, you can navigate the journey towards balance, supporting each other in achieving personal and collective transformation.

For Individual Reflection: If your journey through "Imbalance" is a personal endeavor, this book serves as a reflective companion. Through introspective exercises, examine your own life, identify areas of imbalance, and contemplate actionable steps towards achieving a more balanced existence.

JOURNAL

www.ingramcontent.com/pod-product-compliance
Lightning Source LLC
Chambersburg PA
CBHW051005140626
46546CB00016B/878